Natália Fenner Pena

Phase Angle, Nutritional Status and Clinical Outcomes In Oncology

Natália Fenner Pena

Phase Angle, Nutritional Status and Clinical Outcomes in Oncology

Association of Phase Angle with Nutritional Status and Clinical Outcomes in Surgical Oncology Patients

ScienciaScripts

Imprint

Any brand names and product names mentioned in this book are subject to trademark, brand or patent protection and are trademarks or registered trademarks of their respective holders. The use of brand names, product names, common names, trade names, product descriptions etc. even without a particular marking in this work is in no way to be construed to mean that such names may be regarded as unrestricted in respect of trademark and brand protection legislation and could thus be used by anyone.

Cover image: www.ingimage.com

This book is a translation from the original published under ISBN 978-613-9-60725-9.

Publisher:
Sciencia Scripts
is a trademark of
Dodo Books Indian Ocean Ltd. and OmniScriptum S.R.L publishing group

120 High Road, East Finchley, London, N2 9ED, United Kingdom
Str. Armeneasca 28/1, office 1, Chisinau MD-2012, Republic of Moldova, Europe
Printed at: see last page
ISBN: 978-620-7-30254-3

ACKNOWLEDGEMENTS

First of all, I would like to thank God, my faithful friend, the master of my life... for opening the door, enabling me, enlightening me, not letting me give up, leading me and strengthening me at all times.

To my family. Especially my mum, dad, my brothers, Lipe, Jairo, my mother-in-law Lúcia, grandma Marina and my beloved husband, Leonardo. Thank you for all your unconditional love, your understanding of my frequent absences and your support. Thank you for your encouragement and for always believing in me. You undoubtedly add up to joy, agape love and blessing in my life.

To Professor Dr Simone de Vasconcelos Generoso, my advisor, and to Professor Maria Isabel T D. Correia, my co-supervisor, for the opportunity to do this project, for the learning and growth I have gained in this new challenge and for all the contributions to my scientific training.

To Ariene, my doctoral student, for all her patience, teaching and affection. I can't thank her enough for all the availability (including weekends, evenings and holidays) and knowledge I gained in statistics. I wish you every success and that all your dreams come true! Thank you so much!

To the researchers already involved in this project and to the undergraduate students, especially Nayhara and Regiane. Thank you for going all the way with me to the end of this project, with great determination, so that it could really become a reality. Thank you for your affection, willingness and commitment. I wish you all your dreams come true!

To the coordinators (Professor Aline), teachers and collegiate staff (Mateus) of the Postgraduate Programme in Nutrition and Health at UFMG. I would like to thank Professor Tatiani for her initial receptiveness. Professor Mariza, thank you for your support, even when you were ill, you always welcomed me with a smile on your face, affection and willingness! My thanks also go to Petterson, a professor at the UNA University Centre, for spreading the word and for his support. Thank you all for always adding to and contributing to my education.

To Silvia Maurício, PhD student. Thank you for your teachings, words and patience, which were crucial during the final stretch of this project. Success on your journey!

To my friends and colleagues at the Advanced Heart Institute and Diabetes Weekend Colony (especially Dr Felipe Prado, Physiotherapist Juliano, Dr Levimar Rocha) and Dr Jáder Benedito. Thank you for your clinical contributions, your trust, for supporting me, opening doors, understanding and always cheering me on.

To my prayer group, the small fraternity Casa de Nazaré from the parish of Castelo. Thank you for your prayers, light, strength and friendship! God has guided friends who have strengthened me. Also to Dr Filó, for her words, which were often sudden, but which filled me with hope and made me realise that I don't need to understand or know everything... but that I must do my part, work hard, study hard and only trust, surrender and wait on the Father.

To my friends Mara, Thaís and Karla Canaã for their constant support, prayers and positive energy. Elândia, Gisele, Isabela, Eloisa, my fellow Master's students, thank you for helping me when I needed it and for turning this time together into friendship, with moments of joy and faith. Also to all my colleagues from the first class of the Master's programme in Nutrition and Health.

To the staff at the Hospital das Clínicas (Alfa Institute), especially the nursing team who believed in me and helped me with the blood glucose collection (especially Jane and Nilza). Thank you for your willingness to help, for contributing to this project and for always being willing to help.

To the patients and their families, the subject of this study, who, even with the diagnosis of such a serious illness, showed the courage to face treatment.

In short, it would be impossible to mention everyone here and even unfair to forget anyone... My sincere thanks go to all my friends, colleagues and angels that God has placed in my path during this period.

SUMMARY

Standardised Phase Angle (SFA) is a measurement derived from Electrical Bioimpedance (EBI) adjusted for gender and age. AFP is capable of assessing the integrity of cell membranes and has recently been studied as a possible indicator of nutritional status (NS) and a prognostic factor in cancer patients. However, few studies have assessed the behaviour of AFP as an indicator of nutritional status and adverse clinical outcomes in cancer patients. **Objective: To** assess the association between AFP and preoperative nutritional status variables and clinical outcomes in oncological surgical patients. **Methods: A** longitudinal-prospective study of oncological surgical patients admitted to the Alfa Institute of Gastroenterology at the Hospital das Clínicas in Belo Horizonte, Minas Gerais. Patients' nutritional status was assessed before surgery (preoperative) and clinical outcomes were assessed postoperatively until hospital discharge. Data on nutritional status (NS) was obtained in the immediate preoperative period using the Subjective Global Assessment (SGA), arm circumference (AC), triceps skinfold (TSF), arm muscle area (AMA), weight loss percentage (WLP) and functionality using dynamometry. AFP was obtained using BIA and calculated according to the following equation: AFP=measured AF - mean AF (for age and sex)/standard deviation of the population, according to age and sex. Data on clinical outcomes and capillary glycaemia were collected from medical records and bed runs. Descriptive and bivariate analyses were carried out; agreement between methods using the kappa coefficient and simple logistic regression models were used to assess the association between AFP, nutritional status and clinical outcomes in this population. The Ancova test was used to compare capillary glycaemia means according to AFP categorisation. A significance level of 5% (p<0.05) was adopted for all analyses. **Results:** 121 patients were included in this study. The mean age of the participants was 58.8 ± 12.5 years, and 52.9 per cent were male. The prevalence of malnutrition found according to the AGS was 63.6 per cent, while 28.1 per cent of the patients had AFP values below the 5th percentile. Preoperatively, individuals classified as being at nutritional risk according to the AFP categorisation were more likely to be malnourished according to the AGS (OR=3.66; 95% CI:1.35-9.90), CB (OR=4.24; 95% CI: 1.72-10.43), AMB (OR=4.38; 95% CI: 1.68-11.42), dynamometry (OR=3.84; 95% CI: 1.31-11.25) and having a higher percentage of weight loss (PPP); (OR=3.86; 95% CI: 1.64-9.06); (p<0.05). Significant agreement was observed in the preoperative period between the AFP and AGS classification (0.29; p=0.001), dynamometry (0.25; p=0.003) and AMB (0.24; p=0.003). With regard to clinical outcomes, a high prevalence of infectious complications (57.0%) was identified in the cancer patients assessed, and those classified as being at risk by the AFP were 3.51 (95% CI: 1.37-8.99; p=0.009) times more likely to have infectious complications during their hospital stay. There was no association between AFP and the other outcomes assessed (p>0.05). **Conclusion:** Our findings suggest that the AFP can be considered a useful tool that is earlier than traditional parameters and can help assess and classify the nutritional status of cancer patients in hospital. It also proved to be a good prognostic indicator, capable of predicting infectious complications and showed a significant trend of association in relation to the hospital hyperglycaemia assessed. Future studies could confirm these findings and whether the AFP, used in combination with other nutritional diagnostic tools in these patients, would increase its sensitivity in detecting more debilitated nutritional states.

Keywords: Cancer. Nutritional Status. Standardised Phase Angle. Clinical Outcome. Hospital hyperglycaemia. Muscle Strength.

SUMMARY

CHAPTER 1

INTRODUCTION

Nutritional assessment in the hospital environment still lacks a single method, considered a "standard", which enables the diagnosis of nutritional alterations to be made objectively and with a high level of efficacy, sensitivity and specificity during hospitalisation, especially in cancer patients (ACUNA; CRUZ, 2004; GUPTA *et al.*, 2004a; 2004b).

Phase Angle (PA) has aroused interest in recent decades because it is an objective, fast and non-invasive method obtained using Electrical Bioimpedance (BIA). This parameter derives directly from the relationship between reactance (resistive capacitance of cell membranes) and resistance (pure opposition of the biological conductor to electric current), which body tissues offer to the passage of low-intensity electric current (BARBOSA-SILVA *et al.*, 2005a; NORMAN et *al.*, 2006; BARBOSA-SILVA *et al.*, 2008; PAIVA *et al.*, 2010).

Since PA is capable of reflecting the integrity of cell membranes and water distribution between the intra- and extracellular environment, it has been interpreted as an indicator of health status and is considered a good prognostic marker in various types of pathologies (SCHWENK *et al.*, 2000; SELBERG *et al.*, 2002; KYLE et *al.*, 2012; BERBIGIER et *al.*, 2013), including cancer (GUPTA *et al.*, 2004b; GUPTA *et al.*, 2008; HUI et *al.*, 2014). In addition, evidence has suggested that PA is also associated with changes in nutritional status and can be used as a tool for nutritional diagnosis (BARBOSA-SILVA *et al.*, 2005b; NORMAN *et al.*, 2012; MALECKA-MASSALSKA., 2015).

However, there is still controversy over the use of PA to diagnose nutritional status and predict complications. Much of this disagreement is due to the different cut-off points used in the literature, associated with the fact that PA changes according to some of its determinants, such as gender, age and in different populations (BARBOSA-SILVA, 2008; NORMAN *et al.*, 2012).

In this sense, the use of the Standardised Phase Angle (SPA) has been increasingly proposed (BARBOSA-SILVA, 2008), since this parameter provides the value of the phase angle corrected by the standard deviation determined for the population, according to the patient's age and sex (BARBOSA-SILVA, 2008). According to Paiva *et al.* (2010), PFA is considered an independent prognostic factor in cancer patients for clinical outcomes and survival. In addition, although there are still few studies in the scientific literature, data shows that AFP also seems to be a good marker of nutritional status, providing better prognostic information about individuals than using PA in its absolute values, i.e. obtained in degrees (BARBOSA-SILVA, 2008; PAIVA *et al.,* 2010).

Deterioration and difficulty in maintaining adequate nutritional status are common in hospitalised patients and are directly related to the effectiveness of treatment and quality of life (LEANDRO-MERHI, 2008; KAISER *et al.,* 2010; KVAMME et *al.,* 2015; CACCIALANZA *et al.,* 2015). Cancer patients are known to be at greater risk of malnutrition and post-operative complications (BOZZETTI *et al.,* 2001; 1999; INCA, 2015a). Therefore, nutritional assessment and early interventions are essential in the care of these patients.

Cancer is considered a chronic, non-communicable disease whose main characteristic is disorganised cell growth. It is one of the main causes of death worldwide and is a clear public health problem (GUERRA; GALLO; MENDONÇA, 2005; INCA, 2015a). According to the World Health Organisation (WHO), it is estimated that in 2030 there will be around 21.4 million new cases of cancer and 13.2 million deaths from cancer worldwide (WORLD HEALTH ORGANISATION, 2015).

Around 20 to 62% of hospitalised cancer patients are at risk of malnutrition in countries such as Brazil and approximately 80% of patients admitted to in-hospital services are already in some degree of malnutrition at the time of initial diagnosis (DUCHINI *et al.,* 2010; DUVAL *et al.,* 2010; BADIA-TAHULL *et al.,* 2014). In the study by Azevedo *et al,* 2006), the researchers checked the nutritional status of hospitalised patients and found that malnutrition was present in 24.3% of patients, and when stratified by those diagnosed with cancer, the percentage more than doubled, totalling 53.3% of patients, i.e. just over half of the population assessed. According to data from the Brazilian Oncological Nutrition Survey (IBNO) (INCA, 2013), the prevalence of malnutrition in cancer patients, when assessed by the Global Assessment Produced by the Patient (AGS-PPP), was also high, as around 45.1% of patients were classified with some degree of malnutrition when assessed using this parameter. In a multicentre study carried out with 4,000 hospitalised patients by the Brazilian Nutritional Assessment Survey (IBRANUTRI), it was observed that 48.1% of individuals were classified as malnourished by the Subjective Global Assessment (SGA). The incidence of complications and the mortality rate were, respectively, 11 per cent and 7.7 per cent higher in patients diagnosed with malnutrition when compared to nourished patients. This study also showed that the frequency of severe malnutrition in cancer patients was almost double that observed in the general population (23.3% *vs.* 12.4%). Thus, given the high prevalence of malnutrition, often associated with adverse outcomes still observed in the hospice environment, nutritional assessment is becoming a greater challenge and requires more sensitive and objective methods in order to diagnose increasingly early changes in nutritional status, especially in cancer patients, in order to optimise resources, improve nutritional support and monitoring and, consequently, the quality of life of these individuals.

It has also been shown that hyperglycaemia is a common outcome observed in hospitalised patients and is considered a marker of poor prognosis for critically ill patients, both clinical and surgical (RODRIGUES, 2008). According to Baldasso *et al.* (2006), hyperglycaemia can be triggered by reasons very characteristic of the hospital routine and one of the main causes is stress, which is probably due to an excess release of endogenous hormones. According to the work of Grassani (2011), in the last decade the importance of glycaemic control in the hospital environment has been highlighted, based on the pathophysiology of cellular glucotoxicity, through which it has been possible to better understand the deleterious impact of hyperglycaemia on hospitalised patients and, epidemiologically, to show a strong association between hyperglycaemia, mortality and adverse outcomes. Furthermore, the importance of intensive glycaemic control in hospital settings has become a major focus of recent clinical trials (VAN DER BERGHE *et al.*, 2001; VAN DER BERGHE *et al.*, 2006; GRASSANI, 2011).

In view of the above, the importance of glycaemic assessment in cancer patients is highlighted, in order to verify whether there are significant changes in relation to the times of hospitalisation, the time in which these changes occur and whether this correlates with the phase angle. To date, this is the first study to assess the association between AFP values and capillary glycaemia measurements in cancer patients. Since it would be a plausible hypothesis to investigate the integrity of the cell membrane, as assessed by AFP, and its possible relationship with cellular glycotoxicity caused by the presence of hyperglycaemia.

In this context, this study aimed to assess the nutritional status of surgical oncology patients hospitalised at the Alfa Institute of Gastroenterology, with the main objective of verifying cell integrity using the Standardised Phase Angle (SPA) and comparing it with other parameters routinely used in the nutritional assessment of these patients, as well as evaluating the association of SPA with adverse clinical outcomes and hospital hyperglycaemia.

CHAPTER 2

LITERATURE REVIEW

2.1 Nutritional assessment

Nutritional assessment can be carried out using various instruments, including electrical bioimpedance (BIA), subjective global assessment (SGA) and anthropometric, functional and biochemical parameters (BARBOSA-SILVA; BARROS, 2002; DUCHINI *et al.*, 2010). Each method has advantages and disadvantages (WAITZBERG; CORREIA, 2003) which should be considered according to the population to be assessed and the resources available in each institution.

According to the National Consensus on Oncological Nutrition, developed by the National Cancer Institute (INCA, 2009), the joint use of different nutritional assessment methods in the hospital environment is an important tool, since it covers different data needed for therapy and dietetics. Nutritional care for patients diagnosed with cancer should be individualised and include different types of care up to outpatient follow-up, with the primary aim of preventing or reversing the decline in nutritional status, as well as avoiding the progression of the disease to cachexia, with increased proteolysis and immune response in these patients (INCA, 2013). In this context, the assessment and general nutritional monitoring of cancer patients are fundamental tools that form part of the systematisation of care for hospitalised patients and also aim to achieve better post-surgical results and a better quality of life for these patients (DAVIES, 2005; INCA, 2013).

In hospitalised oncology patients, nutritional assessment is considered to be an even greater challenge, since these patients can present alterations in the balance of body fluids, such as oedema and hyperhydration, directly influencing anthropometric assessment and biochemical tests (FONTES, 2011). Nevertheless, frequent loss and variation in body weight is common and continues to be an important indicator for assessing nutritional status in these patients (RAVASCO *et al.*, 2011). Current studies have shown that weight loss in cancer patients can exceed 10 per cent of body weight during treatment, and that a loss of more than 20 per cent of the patient's total body weight results in increased toxicity and mortality, as well as longer treatment times (PAIXÃO, GONZALEZ and ITO, 2015; COLASANTO *et al.*, 2005). In addition, involuntary weight loss of between 5% and 10% of usual weight can be considered significant and indicates nutritional risk, as well as being directly related to poor prognosis in cancer patients (BOTTONI, 2001). It should be noted that the AGS questionnaire, which includes the Weight Loss Percentage (WLP), despite being considered the gold standard for the nutritional diagnosis of hospitalised patients, because it is subjective, is not considered a sensitive tool for monitoring the nutritional evolution of these individuals (STEENSON; VIVANTI; ISENRING, 2013).

In this sense, there is still no single standardised nutritional assessment method that can be used to monitor the nutritional evolution of patients in hospital. In the absence of a single parameter, joint assessment has been advocated, as it allows for better diagnosis and monitoring of the hospitalised patient's nutritional status (BARBOSA-SILVA *et al.*, 2003; KYLE *et al*, 2004a; MARTINS, 2008; JENSEN *et al.*, 2013; MAULDIN; O'LEARY-KELLEY, 2015).

2.1.1 *Electrical bioimpedance*

Electrical bioimpedance analysis (BIA) is a non-invasive, objective, portable method used to assess body composition through the application of low-intensity electrical current. It is characterised by being a safe method, whose results are reproducible, quick to obtain and reflect the electrical properties of normal or affected tissues and the level of body hydration (BARBOSA-SILVA, 2005; PAIVA, 2007; OLIVEIRA, 2012; PAIXÃO; GONZALEZ; ITO, 2015).

The basic principle of BIA is based on the fact that the human body is made up of a set of five cylinders (two arms, two legs and a torso) that offer different resistances to the passage of low-intensity electric current and that tissue hydration is stable (HORIE *et al.*, 2008). Furthermore, it can be inferred that the human body is divided into two large compartments: one in which most of the body is made up of water and electrolytes, and the other made up of fat and tissues that do not contain water (KYLE *et al*, 2004a). Based on the measurement of the body's total resistance to the passage of low amplitude (500 to 800 AU) and high frequency (50 kHz) electric current, it is possible to identify the main components of BIA: Reactance (Xc), Resistance (R), Impedance (Z) (BARBOSA-SILVA, 2005; HORIE *et al.*, 2008; WILHELM-LEEN *et al.*, 2014; SILVA et *al.*, 2015).

The Reactance measurement (Xc=opposition to the flow of electric current caused by the capacitance produced by the cell membrane) is also related to the extra and intracellular water balance and to the ability of lean tissues to conduct electric current, as they contain a greater amount of water and electrolytes. They therefore present low resistance to the passage of electric current (HORIE *et al.*, 2008). In turn, the measure of Resistance (R=measure of opposition to the flow of electric current through the body) refers to the fat and bone compartments which, because they are not good conductors of energy, offer greater resistance to the passage of this current (KYLE *et al.*, 2004a; KAMIMURA et *al.*, 2005; HORIE et *al.*, 2008). Impedance (Z) is expressed as the square root of the sum of the squares of R and Xc, associated with the circuit, and can also be defined as the drop in voltage when an electric current passes through the body (KYLE *et al.*, 2004a; HORIE *et al.*, 2008).

Different mathematical formulae have been developed from the reactance and resistance values in order to obtain the final result of the amount of body fat, total water and lean muscle mass of individuals (BARBOSA-SILVA, 2005; HORIE *et al.*, 2008).

Different BIA devices can be used. They differ in terms of cost, type of current and frequency, as well as the formulas provided (HORIE *et al.*, 2008). Single-frequency devices (BIA-FU) generally have a frequency of 50kHz, allowing them to estimate fat-free mass (FFM) and provide measurements such as total body water (TBA), but they are unable to distinguish between the distribution of extra- and intracellular water. On the other hand, multi-frequency BIA devices (BIA-MF) are capable of estimating FFM and TCA, differentiating between intra- and extracellular water using different frequencies that can operate from 0 to 1000kHz. Assessment using segmented BIA (BIA- SG) is able to estimate body fat (BF) and lean mass (LBM) by body region, as well as checking for changes in body fluids in different pathologies. It is generally carried out by means of BIA-MF with the addition of 02 electrodes on the wrist and foot, with a view to greater precision in assessing body composition (KYLE *et al.*, 2004a; HORIE *et al.*, 2008).

To perform BIA, the individual must be lying down, with limbs in abduction, arms 30° apart from the trunk and legs 45° apart. Two electrodes are then placed on each limb (one distal and one proximal) unilaterally on the wrist and ankle, with at least 5cm between them (KYLE *et al.*, 2004a). In addition, some recommendations should be followed in order to minimise possible interference in the results, such as: fasting from food, drink and alcohol for at least four hours; skin conditions (the professional carrying out the test should assess the absence of lesions on the patient's skin and at the electrode positioning site, as well as sanitising with alcohol for asepsis); environmental factors (making sure the patient is in a neutral environment, with no contact with the metal of the bed or any other electro or magnetic field. These and other requirements should be adopted before the test begins (KYLE *et al.*, 2004a).

There are some limitations to the use of BIA. The presence of abnormalities in the body composition of some individuals, such as oedema, ascites and general changes in hydration status, can overestimate the value of lean mass (BARBOSA-SILVA *et al.*, 2008;

HORIE *et al.,* 2008). Furthermore, the application and use of standardised formulas or equations found in different types of BIA devices are often only applicable to healthy, eutrophic individuals or specific populations. For this reason, they would not be suitable for assessing all types of study populations (COPPINI *et al.,* 2005; HORIE *et al.,* 2008).

However, BIA can be used more effectively and reliably by using the absolute resistance and reactance values provided directly by the device, without the need to use formulas, weight or specific regression equations. One way of using these values is to obtain the Phase Angle, which is derived directly from the relationship between resistance and reactance (KYLE *et al.,* 2004b; BARBOSA-SILVA, 2005) and appears to be related to malnutrition and nutritional post-intervention (BARBOSA-SILVA., 2003; NORMAN *et al.,* 2006; MALECKA-MASSALSKA., 2015).

2.1.2 Phase Angle (PA)

The Phase Angle (PA) determined by BIA analysis is derived directly from the relationship between the Reactance (Xc: resistive capacitance of cell membranes) and Resistance (R: pure opposition of the biological conductor to the electric current) (FIGURE 1) offered by body tissues, and is interpreted as an indicator of cell membrane integrity, as well as being related to prognosis and the patient's general state of health (NORMAN *et al.,* 2006; PAIVA *et al.,* 2010).

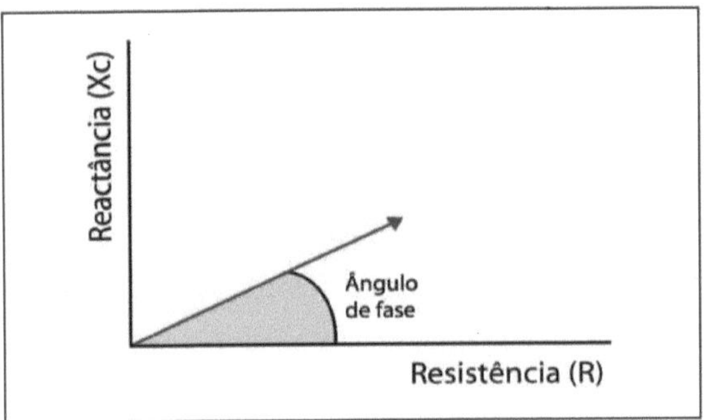

Figure 1 - Electrical and physical properties of BIA: formation of the Phase Angle

Source: Adapted figure. Prepared by the author, based on Ganep (2015).

The AF is the angle formed by the deviation of the electric current that is applied to the body, created when this current crosses the cell membranes, part of which will store energy, acting as capacitors. This creates a phase change, geometrically generating the angular transformation of capacitance or the so-called AF (BARBOSA-SILVA, 2003; BARBOSA-SILVA *et al.,* 2005a).

AF can be obtained using the following equation: AF= arc tangent Xc/R x 180°/ π where π pi= 3.1416 (BARBOSA-SILVA *et al.*, 2005a; BARBOSA- SILVA *et al.*, 2008). Changes in reactance indicate alterations in the patient's cellular integrity or changes in membrane permeability or cellular composition. The more intact the membranes, the greater the energy storage and, consequently, the greater the PA formed (BARBOSA-SILVA *et al.*, 2005a; KYLE et *al.*, 2012).

AF can vary from zero degrees (system without cell membranes, resistive) to ninety degrees (system without fluids, only capacitive). Healthy individuals have average PA values of between 4 and 15 degrees. The variation in PA depends on the age and sex of the individual (BARBOSA-SILVA, 2008), tissue cellularity, tissue hydration and membrane permeability, which can be altered by the disease process itself (BARBOSA- SILVA, 2005; SILVA: CARUSO; MARTINI, 2007; BARBOSA-SILVA *et al.*, 2008; MOTTA et *al.*, 2015).

By definition, PA is positively associated with reactance and negatively associated with resistance (MALECKA-MASSALSKA *et al.*, 2015). Lower AF indicates cell death or a decline in the cellular integrity of individuals, while high phase angles indicate a greater amount of intact cell membranes (SELBERG *et al.*, 2002).

In addition, PA is also associated with a reduction in body cell mass, reflecting disturbances in the electrical properties of normal or affected tissues, and the level of body hydration, which changes in different diseases (BARBOSA-SILVA., 2008; KYLE *et al.*, 2004a; EICKEMBERG *et al.*, 2011; BERBIGIER et *al.*, 2013; LLAMES *et al.*, *2013*). According to BARBOSA-SILVA (2008), malnutrition could be detected earlier by changes in the cell membrane and the imbalance of body fluids.

Studies in the literature (BARBOSA-SILVA *et al.*, 2003; NORMAN et *al.*, 2006; BARBOSA-SILVA *et al.*, 2008; PAIVA *et al.*, 2011; BERBIGIER *et al.*, 2013; PAIXÃO; GONZALEZ, 2015) indicate that PA seems to be a marker of the nutritional status of hospitalised patients.

Selberg *et al.* (2002) assessed PA in a heterogeneous group of 1,035 hospitalised patients (589 of whom were men) and the mean PA value found was 4.9°. This value was significantly lower than that observed in healthy individuals (4.9° *vs.* 6.6°; p<0.001). Gupta *et al.* (2008) assessed the relationship between PA and nutritional status, as diagnosed by AGS, in patients with advanced colorectal cancer. The results showed that in well-nourished patients, mean PA was significantly higher (6.12°) compared to those who were malnourished (5.18°). The authors concluded that PA is a nutritional indicator in patients diagnosed with colorectal cancer, but report that more research is needed to clarify the ideal cut-off point in order to be incorporated for better nutritional assessment.

In a more recent study of cancer patients undergoing pre-radiotherapy, Motta *et al.* (2015) showed that the PA cut-off point of 5.2 degrees or 5.4 degrees was suitable for assessing nutritional status compared to BMI and SFA, respectively.

PA has also been reported in the literature as a good prognostic indicator in relation to disease progression, incidence of post-operative complications and length of hospital stay (NORMAN *et al.*, 2010; HUI *et al.*, 2014), as well as an indicator of survival in patients with colorectal cancer (Gupta et *al.* 2008; with pancreatic cancer (GUPTA et *al.*, 2004b), and in patients diagnosed with lung cancer (TOSO *et al.*, 2000). Thus, low PA values are associated with disease progression and negative clinical outcomes (NORMAN *et al.*, 2010).

Gupta *et al.* (2008) evaluated the prognostic role of PA in patients with advanced colorectal cancer. The authors observed that patients with PA < 5.7° had a lower average survival (95% CI: 4.8-12.4 months; n=26), compared to patients with PA > 5.57°, who had a higher average survival (95% CI: 21.9-58.8 months; n=26), (p<0.0001). In another study carried out by the group with 58 patients diagnosed with pancreatic cancer, it was observed that patients with PA values <5° had a mean survival time of 6.3 months, while patients with PA >5° had a superior survival (10.2 months); (p<0.02). These results suggest PA as a prognostic indicator in patients with advanced pancreatic cancer. However, more research is needed with a larger number of participants and in different pathologies in order to establish the real value of this marker (GUPTA *et al.*, 2004a).

One of the advantages of using HF is that it is independent of regression equations and the individual's weight, and therefore allows the patient to be assessed using direct measurements of reactance and resistance. Thus, PA could be used in patients in whom anthropometry cannot be measured or in situations in which it is not appropriate to use the equations inserted into the BIA device (NAGANO; SUITA; YAMANOUCHI, 2000; BARBOSA-SILVA *et al.*, 2003; GUPTA *et al.*, 2004a; 2004b; MIKA et *al.*, 2004; BARBOSA-SILVA *et al.*, 2005b). It should also be noted that most authors have used and generated PA cut-off points in degrees within the study population. This is one of the disadvantages of using this method (BARBOSA-SILVA, 2005a; 2008), since these cut-off points are not necessarily applicable to other populations and in different clinical contexts (NORMAN *et al.*, 2010).

It should be noted that the studies available on cancer patients on the predictive value of cell function indicators derived from the electrical and biological properties of tissues are still scarce (BARBOSA-SILVA, 2003; NORMAN *et al.*, 2006; CASTANHO *et al.*, 2013).

To date, around 30 publications are available on the PubMed scientific database, relating PA to nutritional status, electrical bioimpedance and cancer. Furthermore, like any biological marker, PA can change and be influenced according to different determinants, such as population, age and gender (BARBOSA-SILVA *et al.*, 2008), and the use of AFP (Standardised Phase Angle) is indicated instead of its measurement in degrees, i.e. its absolute value (PAIVA *et al.*, 2011).

2.1.3 *The Standardised Phase Angle (SPA)*

The Standardised Phase Angle (SFA) refers to the mean values of the standard deviation of the adjusted phase angle for a given population, according to age and sex. It is obtained by subtracting the expected average PA value for a given population from the measured PA value and dividing by the standard deviation (according to the reference values determined for that same population, according to age group and gender) (BARBOSA-SILVA *et al.*, 2005b; BARBOSA-SILVA *et al.*, 2008).

Reference values for standardising the phase angle were presented for the healthy American, German, Swiss and Brazilian populations, in order to also adjust the values according to the individual's sex and age group. Lower PA values were observed in female patients, due to the smaller amount of muscle mass present, and also in the elderly, probably due to the reduction in body cell mass resulting from the ageing process itself (BARBOSA-SILVA *et al.*, 2005a; BARBOSA-SILVA; BARROS, 2005; BOSY- WESTPHAL *et al.*, 2006; BARBOSA-SILVA *et al.*, 2008; LLAMES et *al.*, 2013).

In a study of 399 cancer patients, Norman *et al.* (2010) found that 78% of the patients who had an AFP lower than the fifth percentile were diagnosed with moderate or severe malnutrition using the AGS, compared to patients who had higher AFP values (39.1%; p<0.05).

In another study, Paiva *et al.* (2011) found that AFP adjusted according to gender and age based on the reference values for the Brazilian population, according to the classification by Barbosa-Silva *et al.* (2008), was an independent prognostic indicator for clinical complications and mortality rates in cancer patients undergoing chemotherapy. According to this study, the cut-off point corresponding to -1.65 would represent the 5th percentile and could be considered the lower limit accepted for the healthy population (PAIVA *et al.*, 2010). In this way, the AFP could be used to compare studies of different populations, genders and ages.

Considering that there are still few studies in the scientific literature, these data seem to demonstrate the usefulness of AFP as a more objective marker in assessing the nutritional status of hospitalised patients, as well as a good predictor, capable of providing better clinical and prognostic information (BARBOSA-SILVA *et al.* 2008; PAIVA *et al.*, 2010).

2.1.4 Subjective Global Assessment (SGA)

The Subjective Global Assessment (SGA) was developed in 1982 and validated in 1987. It is considered to be an essentially clinical nutritional assessment tool (DETSKY *et al.*, 1987).

It is considered a simple, low-cost, non-invasive, easy-to-perform assessment method that can be applied at the patient's bedside. This method was initially developed and validated for hospitalised surgical patients, but it is also well accepted in different clinical situations and is considered a reference tool in nutritional assessment (DETSKY *et al.*, 2008).

The AGS is good at diagnosing nutritional status, as well as predicting the risk of complications and mortality (BARBOSA-SILVA; BARROS, 2006). Given these facts, in recent decades the AGS has been successfully reproduced in clinical practice and in hospital settings, as well as in research with different groups of patients (WAITZBERG; CAIAFFA; CORREIA, 2001; BARBOSA-SILVA; BARROS, 2006; DETSKY *et al.*, 2008).

The assessment is carried out using a wide-ranging form that covers the main characteristics such as: weight loss in the last six months and PPP, changes in the patient's food intake, the presence of gastrointestinal symptoms, changes in functional capacity, physical aspects and the metabolic demand of the disease, the latter being classified as mild, moderate or severe (DETSKY *et al.*, 1987; BOTTONI, 2001). Changes in food intake are assessed according to the patient's habits and include issues such as: fasting, type of diet (liquid, pasty and solid diet) in a reduced quantity than usual. Gastrointestinal symptoms include the presence of nausea, vomiting and/or diarrhoea in the last two weeks. Functional capacity is related to the ability to carry out daily or routine physical activities, such as doing household chores or even working. With regard to the physical examination, loss of subcutaneous fat (triceps and subscapular region), muscle depletion, presence of oedema (usually in the ankle and sacral region) and ascites should be assessed. After the assessment, patients are classified as nourished, suspected malnourished, moderately malnourished or severely malnourished.

According to Correia *et al.* (1998), the accuracy of the method depends on important factors such as clinical experience, technique and, above all, the adequate training of health professionals in order to achieve good agreement between different evaluators.

However, the AGS has some limitations, such as not being considered a monitoring parameter during hospitalisation, since it does not have adequate sensitivity to detect small changes in the nutritional status of cancer patients (STEENSON; VIVANTI; ISENRING,2013).

For specific use in oncological patients, Ottery (1996) adapted the AGS with the main alterations observed in these patients and named it the Patient-Produced Subjective Global Assessment of Nutritional Status (PG-SGA). This was validated and translated into Portuguese (GONZALEZ., 2009). It should be emphasised that this assessment differs from the original in three main aspects: a more specific assessment of the symptoms of nutritional impact present in cancer patients, such as dry mouth, the presence of a metallic taste, among others. The second aspect is related to the transformation of the score into scores, thus allowing for a more objective assessment, with cut-off points that allow for different levels of nutritional interventions (INCA., 2013). Lastly, the AGS-PPP has the main objective of allowing greater participation by the patient themselves, where it covers more answers to questions such as weight loss at different times and more specific symptoms (GONZALEZ, 2009; INCA., 2013). However, in public hospitals, its use and implementation is very limited due to the level of education and culture of most patients, as well as the need for adequate training for professionals. In this context, it can be seen that we still don't have a single objective, consistent and standard tool for the nutritional diagnosis of oncological patients in the hospital environment. To compound this problem, there is a lack of universal agreement on the definition and validation of nutritional assessment indicators in hospitals (MALECKA-MASSALSKA *et al.*, 2015). However, even though the AGS and AGS-PPP have some limitations related to subjectivity, they are validated tools that are still widely used and indicated for predicting a reduction in the quality of life of these patients, usually associated with some method of nutritional assessment, such as anthropometry.

2.1.5 Anthropometry

Anthropometry is used to measure body weight, girth and skinfold thickness. It is considered a simple and low-cost method (ROCHE; MARTORELL, 1988; LOHMAN, 1992; CALIXTO-LIMA, GONZALEZ, 2013).

Body weight expresses the size of the body's mass or volume, i.e. it represents the sum of all the body's components (water, fat, bones and muscles). However, weight should be used and interpreted with caution, especially when the individual has alterations, such as water retention (oedema or ascites) and signs of dehydration. It is therefore not indicated as a single, isolated measure when assessing the nutrition of hospitalised patients (DUERKSEN *et al.*, 2000; DEURENBERG, 2003).

Involuntary weight change is important information used to assess the severity of these individuals' health problems, since weight loss has a high correlation with mortality (KYLE *et al.*, 2004b). Weight loss of more than 10 per cent of the patient's usual weight is related to alterations in the immune system and an increased risk of complications (KYLE *et al.*, 2004b). The ratio of the patient's weight to their height will determine their Body Mass Index (BMI). According to (DEWYS *et al.*, 1980), it has long been known that weight loss is a common condition among cancer patients at the time of initial diagnosis. Involuntary weight loss is generally associated with poor quality of life, poor response to treatment and a high mortality rate (VIGANO *et al.*, 2000).

BMI is based on the relationship between current or estimated weight and height, establishing body weight per height squared in metres (kg/height x height). Values between 18.5 kg/m^2 and 24.9 kg/m^2 are considered normal for healthy adults (WHO, 1997). According to the WHO, BMI is one of the most practical measures used to assess malnutrition and obesity rates in large populations. However, the main limitation of this index is that it does not distinguish muscle mass and fat mass from the individual's total body mass. In other words, it is unable to accurately assess lean mass or adipose tissue or differentiate between them. Given this fact, it is questionable whether it should be used for nutritional assessment in a hospital environment (CALIXTO-LIMA; GONZALEZ, 2013). Furthermore, its interpretation in situations where patients are hyperhydrated, have signs of dehydration, are severely ill or bedridden, should be done with great caution and, in most cases, the use of BMI is even contraindicated, so as not to misclassify the patient's nutritional status (KYLE *et al.*, 2004b).

The arm circumference (AC) measurement represents the sum of the areas made up of bone, fat and muscle tissue in the arm. This measurement is capable of informing about changes in the mass of individuals, however, if used in isolation, the BC is not capable of discerning whether the depletion is muscle or fat mass (LOHMAN; ROCHE; MARTORELL, 1988;HEYMSFIELD *et al.*,1993).

Skinfold assessment is a practical, simple and low-cost method, carried out using a device called a plicometer. Skinfolds are commonly used in clinical practice to assess body fat percentage. The rationale for estimating body fat is based on the fact that approximately half of the body's total fat content is found in the subcutaneous tissue (LOHMAN, 1992; CALIXTO-LIMA; GONZALEZ, 2013). Most protocols for determining body fat by skinfolds use between two and nine measurement sites, depending on the environment to be used and the profile of the individuals being assessed (SIRI, 1961; LOHMAN, 1992; MARFELL-JANES *et al.*, 2006).

The triceps skinfold (TSF) is measured on the upper arm, at the midpoint between the acromion and the olecranon. It is considered the most important fold in clinical practice for classifying a patient's nutritional status, as it is the region most representative of the body's subcutaneous fat reserve, i.e. it is capable of measuring existing fat depletion (LOHMAN, 1992; CALIXTO-LIMA; GONZALEZ, 2013).

The arm muscle area (AMB) can be calculated from the measurement of CB and DCT (HEYMSFIELD *et al.*, 1993; LOHMAN; ROCHE; MARTORELL, 1988).

AMB is a parameter capable of assessing the reserve of muscle tissue, correcting for bone area and relating more adequately to changes in muscle tissue, gauging the existing deficit. It is calculated using mathematical formulae between the ratio of BC and TSD measurements (LOHMAN, 1998; WAITZBERG, 2004; ACUNA; CRUZ, 2004; MUSSOI, 2014).

Some limitations are found in the use of these parameters in nutritional assessment, such as the lack of reference values for certain populations, limitations in relation to the types and calibration of instruments used and also due to the state of body hydration of hospitalised individuals, which is constantly changing. In addition, alterations can occur due to the differences observed in relation to the assessor, who can make mistakes when measuring if they are not well adapted and trained (LOHMAN,1992; RECH, *et al.*, 2010). Therefore, anthropometry should not be used as an isolated parameter in the nutritional assessment of hospitalised patients.

2.1.6 Manual dynamometry

Dynamometry assesses handgrip strength, which is a measure of muscle strength (SCHLUSSEL; ANJOS; KAC, 2008). In order to measure voluntary muscle strength, a simple test is carried out using a device called a dynamometer, in which the capacity and function of the skeletal muscle is estimated using the strength of the hand grip. Although this method is still not widely available in public services and costs relatively more than the usual anthropometric parameters, it is considered cheap, practical and quick, as it can be carried out by any qualified health professional at the patient's bedside (WEBB *et al.*, 1989; MARTINS, 2008; CRUZ-JENTOFT *et al.*, 2010).

Manual dynamometry can be considered an indirect tool for assessing nutritional status since muscle activity is linked to cellular energy functioning, and skeletal muscle function can be rapidly altered in the presence of malnutrition. Thus, before anthropometric changes occur, there are functional changes resulting from the disease itself, such as a decrease in muscle strength (CORREIA, 2001; BUDZIARECK; DUARTE; BARBOSA-SILVA *et al.*, 2008; PASTORES; OEHLSCHALAEGER; GONZALEZ, 2013).

Normam *et al.* (2005) assessed 287 hospitalised individuals and observed that those who were malnourished according to BMI classification had lower muscle strength compared to eutrophic patients. In another study of 189 cancer patients, Norman *et al.* (2010) found that the presence of malnutrition was an independent risk factor for a decline in muscle strength and impaired functional status.

Limberger *et al.* (2014), in a more recent study, assessed 23 cancer patients. The results showed an association between hand grip strength determined by dynamometry and nutritional status, according to the AGS-PPP classification. These findings show that malnutrition is an important factor contributing to reduced muscle function.

However, there are some limitations to the use of dynamometry in relation to the traditional nutritional assessment of hospitalised patients. The lack of equipment due to reduced costs and availability of funds in public hospitals, as well as the lack of experience of qualified professionals with the appropriate technique, could make it difficult to use in this environment (SCHLUSSEL; ANJOS; KAC, 2008). Furthermore, no single global cut-off point has been described. Many reference values available in scientific literature were developed for healthy adults (SCHLUSSEL; ANJOS; KAC, 2008; BUDZIARECK; DUARTE; BARBOSA-SILVA, 2008). The study by Budziareck, Duarte and Barbosa-Silva (2008), carried out with 300 healthy adults aged between 18 and 90 of both sexes, established cut-off points for manual dynamometry, in which values classified below the 5th percentile of reference for the population were considered to be muscle strength depletion.

Chen *et al.* (2011) applied manual dynamometry cut-off values to pre-surgical individuals diagnosed with oesophageal cancer (54 men and 7 women), with an average age of 60.7 years, in which muscle depletion was defined as handgrip strength of less than 25kg. The authors concluded that patients with handgrip strength depletion are at greater risk of complications and that the dynamometry test is cheap, quick and has high predictive power, and can be included in the routine preoperative assessment of cancer patients.

2.2 Cancer and malnutrition

Cancer is the term used to classify a variety of malignant diseases characterised by the abnormal growth of cells (neoplasms). It is considered a chronic, non-transmissible, multifactorial disease that causes mutations in the body, such as uncontrolled and disorganised cell growth, changes in genetic expression associated with metabolic deregulation and an inflammatory state (MORIN *et al.*, 2008; KRAWCZYK *et al.*, 2014). These changes lead to a lack of control in the process of programmed cell death (apoptosis) and cell division (mitosis), which can spread throughout the body from the primary focus, via the lymphatic or blood pathways, causing metastasis (KRAWCZYK *et al.*, 2014; INCA, 2015a).

Cancer is considered the second leading cause of death in the world (INCA, 2015b). The estimate for 2016, which is also valid for 2017, shows that there will be approximately 596,000 new cases of cancer in Brazil. Among men, 295,200 thousand cases are expected and among women, 300,800 thousand cases; reinforcing the magnitude of the problem (INCA, 2015b).

The incidence rates (per 100,000 inhabitants) estimated for 2016 for the most frequent types of cancer in the country show that 16.84 per cent of men suffer from colon and rectal cancer and 13.04 per cent from stomach cancer, with the highest prevalence rates found in the southeast and south of Brazil,

respectively (INCA, 2016). With regard to the location of the tumour in women, the data shows that 17.10% of cases of colon and rectal cancer and 7.37% of stomach cancer occur, with the highest prevalence found in the southern region of the country.

It should be noted that the location of the tumour has a direct impact on the patient's evolution. The presence of tumours in the gastrointestinal tract and attached organs such as the liver and bile ducts can cause obstruction or impair the absorption of nutrients, resulting in severe weight loss and malnutrition (VICENTE *et al.*, 2013).

Malnutrition is a frequent and multifactorial manifestation in cancer patients and is considered one of the main contributors to morbidity and mortality, regardless of tumour type and location (MALECKA-MASSALSKA *et al.*, 2015).

Around 20% to 62% of hospitalised cancer patients are at risk of malnutrition (BRUUN *et al.*, 1999; DUCHINI, *et al;* 2010; DUVAL *et al.*, 2010; BADIA-TAHULL *et al.*, 2014). In a recent study, Fernandéz *et al.* (2014) assessed the nutritional status of 201 patients admitted to a university hospital and found that 50.2 per cent were at nutritional risk and 11.9 per cent were classified as malnourished by the AGS. The highest prevalence of malnutrition was observed in the oncology sector (80.0%). According to data from the Brazilian Oncological Nutrition Survey (INCA, 2013), the prevalence of malnutrition in cancer patients assessed by the AGS-PPP is also high, as around 45.1% of patients were classified with some degree of malnutrition using this parameter.

Malnutrition is also associated with longer hospital stays and a greater likelihood of readmission, causing a negative economic effect with higher costs (WAITZBERG; CAIAFFA; CORREIA, 2001; MARTÍNEZ-OLMOS *et al.*, 2005; CALAZANS *et al.*, 2015). Poor nutritional status also has an impact on mortality, with around 20 per cent of cancer patients dying mainly due to malnutrition (BARBOSA-SILVA *et al.*, 2003; PAIVA *et al.*, 2010; JOSEP-ARGILÉS *et al.*, 2014).

Different factors are involved in the development of malnutrition in cancer patients. Due to the underlying pathology, these individuals have physiological, functional and metabolic alterations caused by the presence of the tumour itself, as well as reduced food intake and increased energy needs due to the presence of the tumour mass itself, as well as the side effects of treatment that have repercussions on alterations in nutritional status, with greater risks of post-operative complications and adverse clinical outcomes (ALLISON., 2000; RAVASCO *et al.*, 2005; SHANG *et al.*, 2006; ISENRING, 2007; COSTA, 2012; LUCAS; FAYH, 2012). Furthermore, psychological factors can interfere with the quality of life of these patients and have a negative impact on appetite and food intake (FERREIRA; SCARPA; SILVA, 2008).

The main metabolic alterations caused by the presence of the tumour are related to changes in carbohydrate metabolism, which include a decrease in glucose tolerance as a result of peripheral tissue resistance to insulin action and changes in the sensitivity of pancreatic beta cells to insulin release (BOZZETTI *et al.*, 2001; EHRMANN-JÓSKO *et al.*, 2006; FAROOKI; SCHNEIDER, 2007; GIBNEY *et al.*, 2007). Hepatic glucose metabolism may also be altered, secondary to an increase in the rate of hepatic glucose production due to increased gluconeogenesis from various precursors such as lactate, alanine and glycerol (BOZZETTI *et al.*, 2001).

These patients also have alterations in lipid and protein metabolism. There is an increase in lipolysis, with a concomitant reduction in fatty acid synthesis due to enzymatic alterations such as lipoprotein lipase. There is also the release of lipolytic tumour factors (BOZZETTI *et al.*, 2001; CERNE *et al.*, 2007) and a decrease in muscle protein synthesis with substantial loss of skeletal muscle. These changes are stimulated by the production and release of inflammatory mediators, such as: tumour necrosis factor alpha (TNF; a cytokine involved in cancer proliferation), interleukins (glycoproteins produced by inflammatory cells in response to stress), specifically interleukin-1 beta (IL-1) and interleukin-6 (IL-6), as well as proteolysis-inducing factor (PIF). Excessive and prolonged secretion of these cytokines leads to adverse effects related to anorexia, for example, and is also associated with tumour progression and muscle protein degradation, with consequent weight loss (BOZZETTI *et al.*, 1992; JANKOWSKA; KOSACKA, 2003, WAITZBERG *et al.*, 2004; JATOI *et al.*, 2006; MELSTROM et *al.*, 2007). In addition, other factors are also associated with malnutrition in these patients, such as the location of the tumour and the stage of the disease. In this sense, patients with advanced cancer tend to have a poorer nutritional status (LIMA; MAIO, 2012).

It is important to note that there are different methods of treatment for cancer, such as surgery, chemotherapy, radiotherapy or bone marrow transplantation. The choice of method will depend on the location of the mass of tumour cells and the doctor-patient approach, in order to control symptoms that may interfere with the quality and survival of the patient (RICHTER *et al.*, 2012; INCA, 2015c). Surgery, considered one of the oldest therapies, remains a mainstay and one of the most efficient methods for treating a variety of neoplasms (CUNNINGHAM *et al.*, 2007; HOFF *et al.*, 2013).

Oncological patients therefore require proper diagnosis and monitoring of their nutritional status. Nutritional assessment should be carried out at the beginning and throughout treatment in order to identify patients who are at nutritional risk or malnourished, so as to start nutritional therapy earlier and minimise or even avoid unfavourable clinical outcomes resulting from the pathology itself or from the surgical process.

2.3 Clinical outcomes and hospital hyperglycaemia

Patients hospitalised with a cancer diagnosis have various consequences related to the pathology itself and changes in nutritional status. These include an increased incidence of complications, length of hospital stay and death (DELGADO-RODRÍGUEZ et *al.*, 2002; PAN *et al.*, 2013).

According to data from the Brazilian Hospital Nutritional Assessment Survey (INCA, 2013), the incidence of complications and the mortality rate were respectively 11% and 7.7% higher in patients diagnosed with malnutrition when compared to well-nourished patients according to the AGS classification (WAITZBERG *et al.*, 2001). Other studies corroborate these findings. Braunschweig, Gomez and Sheean (2000) and Álvarez-Hernández *et al.* (2012) observed that, in hospitalised patients, malnutrition is directly related to length of stay, hospital readmission and mortality. In the study by Chen *et al.* (2011), among the 61 patients hospitalised and assessed for surgical treatment of oesophageal cancer, the presence of complications was observed, such as respiratory failure in twelve patients, pneumonia in seven individuals and five patients with fistula. It should be noted that, in this study, the depletion of handgrip strength assessed was also significantly associated ($p<0.05$) with the mortality rate in the post-surgical period.

Another common and frequent outcome triggered in patients in the hospital environment is hyperglycaemia, in patients with or without a diagnosis of diabetes. Assessing this parameter during hospitalisation is important as it can lead to changes in various organs and systems, such as cardiovascular and cerebrovascular changes, acute renal failure, septicaemia and organ dysfunction, as well as increasing the mortality rate (GRASSANI, 2011). In addition, the deleterious effects of hospital hyperglycaemia can affect and compromise the immunity and healing of patients in the postoperative period, as well as contributing to increased oxidative stress, among other outcomes that lead to an increase in various complications (BONAMICHI *et al.*, 2015).

Different mechanisms have been proposed to explain how hyperglycaemia can cause harm to hospitalised patients. Complications occur mainly due to the appearance of infections, favouring septic states in these patients, the hydroelectrolytic disturbances that are evident, endothelial dysfunction due to the intensified presence of inflammation, secondary thrombotic phenomena, the generation of superoxide radicals and the release of inflammatory cytokines (GRASSANI, 2011). It has also been shown that hyperglycaemia is a marker of poor prognosis for critically ill patients, both clinical and surgical (RODRIGUES, 2008).

According to Baldasso *et al.* (2006), hyperglycaemia can be triggered by different reasons that are very typical of the hospital routine and the main causes are metabolic stress, which is probably due to an excess release of endogenous stress hormones such as glucagon and cortisol, as well as the release of inflammatory cytokines in cases of sepsis or surgical trauma (GOMES *et al.*, 2014).

Hyperglycaemia also indirectly influences cancer cells by increasing the levels of inflammatory cytokines (especially interleukins such as IL-1, IL-6) in insulin circulation and, furthermore, there is reason to infer that hyperglycaemia alone has a direct impact on cancer cell proliferation, apoptosis and metastasis. Elevated blood glucose activates various metabolic signalling pathways that cooperate to control cancer cell behaviour such as proliferation, migration, invasion and recurrence (RYU; PARK; SCHERER, 2014).

According to guidelines from the Brazilian Diabetes Society (SBD) (SOCIEDADE

BRASILEIRA DE DIABETES, 2014), checking blood glucose levels, known as glycaemic monitoring, can be done using blood samples taken from different sites, such as venous, arterial or capillary catheters. Capillary measurement is considered a non-invasive procedure, used in hospital environments and as a routine in clinical practice, due to its easy accessibility and the need for simple training for healthcare professionals, or even at home, by the patients themselves using a device called a glucometer or also by the CGMS system (*Continuous Glucose Monitoring System*), which reads blood glucose levels in real time. However, although the latter shows glycaemic variation in a more complete way over the course of the patient's day, it is known that due to costs, this system is not widely used or available in the public and hospital sector, and it is more appropriate to use a glucometer to measure glycaemia in a more practical and effective way.

Regardless of the previous diagnosis of diabetes, the presence of hyperglycaemia in hospitalised patients and also in the Intensive Care Unit (ICU) is associated with adverse clinical outcomes that may reflect greater severity of the underlying disease. It is known that hyperglycaemia in itself contributes to increasing the severity of any disease and causes glucotoxicity (GOMES *et al.*, 2014).

Cellular glycotoxicity can be interpreted as the presence of chronic hyperglycaemia, which can have deleterious effects on the patient's body, especially on the function of pancreatic beta cells, which are present in the islets of langerhans in the pancreas. These are responsible for synthesising and secreting the hormone insulin, which regulates blood glucose levels (FORCINA; ALMEIDA; RIBEIRO JR, 2008). Glycotoxicity can cause deleterious effects at a cellular level, triggered by hyperglycaemia, as well as different consequences, such as a reduction in glucose tolerance and changes in the sensitivity of beta cells, in addition to their reduction through apoptosis (FORCINA; ALMEIDA; RIBEIRO-JR, 2008). This leads to a lack of glycaemic control which, in the long term, can be toxic to the hospitalised patient's body. This situation usually occurs in the presence of very high blood glucose levels (> 250mg/dl) in which there has been no previous therapeutic intervention or care (RUBINO *et al.*, 2004; FORCINA; ALMEIDA; RIBEIRO JR, 2008). It is also known that an increase in blood glucose activates various signalling pathways that cooperate to control the behaviour of cancer cells, such as proliferation, migration, invasion and recurrence (RYU; PARK; SCHERER, 2014) and that in cancer patients, due to the release of tumour factors (PIF: proteolysis-inducing factor and LMF: lipid-mobilising factor) and pro-inflammatory cytokines (IL-1 and IL-6), changes occur in liver and carbohydrate metabolism, with a significant increase in gluconeogenesis and insulin resistance (UMPIERREZ *et al.*, 2002; WAITZBERG *et al.*, 2004; GRASSANI., 2011). Therefore, glycaemic measurements are also considered an important prognostic factor to be assessed, given the possibility of variability and amplitude of oscillations that exist in the hospital environment and in cancer patients.

In view of the above, the importance of assessing glycaemia in cancer patients before and after surgery is highlighted, in order to check whether there are significant changes in relation to the time of hospitalisation, the time in which these changes occur and whether this correlates with the phase angle.

It should be noted that, to date, this was the first study to assess the association between AFP values and capillary glycaemia measurements in surgical oncology patients, since it would be a plausible hypothesis to investigate the integrity of the cell membrane assessed by AFP and its possible relationship with cellular glycotoxicity caused by the presence of hyperglycaemia in the hospital environment.

CHAPTER 3

OBJECTIVES

3.1 General

To assess the association between AFP and preoperative nutritional status variables and clinical outcomes in oncological surgical patients.

3.2 Specific

- To assess the association between the nutritional status of surgical oncology patients and the location of the tumour, age and gender;
- To assess the agreement between the AFP and the nutritional assessment methods used at the Alfa Institute of Gastroenterology;
- To assess the presence of hyperglycaemia in the hospital environment and its supposed association with AFP at different times during hospitalisation.

CHAPTER 4

METHODS

4.1 Study design and population

This is a prospective observational study carried out at the Alfa Institute of Gastroenterology at the Hospital das Clínicas of the Federal University of Minas Gerais.

The sample consisted of patients aged 18 or over, of both sexes, diagnosed with cancer and admitted to the unit for surgery. All the patients signed the Free and Informed Consent Form (FICF) (APPENDIX A) previously approved by the Research Ethics Committee of the Federal University of Minas Gerais (UFMG) CAEE 12279713.1.0000.5149.

In order to estimate the total sample of participants (n=77), the criteria proposed by Hulley *et al.* (2001) for the comparison test of dependent means were adopted, considering the mean and standard deviation of PA (5.12±0.89) identified in a study with Brazilian cancer patients (PAIVA *et al.*, 2010). As recommended in the literature, an association magnitude of 10%, significance level of 5% and test power of 80% were adopted. A value of 20% was also considered as the percentage of possible data loss (BROWNER; CUMMINGS; HULLEY, 2001). A sub-sample was used for capillary glycaemia. To calculate this sub-sample (n=38), we considered the proportion of 13.5% as the value of hyperglycaemia up to the first 48 days of hospitalisation, as identified in the work by Lucas and Fayh (2012), using a finite population sample of 77 individuals, setting the significance level at 5% (alpha or type I error) and the sampling error at 5%, according to the criteria proposed by Hulley *et al.* (2001).

Individuals with limitations that compromised data collection (neurological sequelae, dystrophy, altered level of consciousness, amputees, those with motor paralyses and pacemakers), pregnant women, nursing mothers and those who refused to sign the informed consent form were excluded from the study.

The patients were assessed at three different times: A) twenty-four hours before the operation (PRE-OP) to assess nutritional status and capillary glycaemia; B) between the third and fifth postoperative day (3rd and 5th postoperative days).

DPO) for capillary glycaemia assessment and C) at hospital discharge, also for capillary glycaemia assessment.

4.2 Data collection

Data was collected using a structured questionnaire (APPENDIX B) covering the following items: patient identification; health history; nutritional assessment and clinical outcome, as described:

4.2.1 Patient identification

Personal information, such as medical record number, contact telephone number, gender, age, date of birth and date of hospitalisation.

4.2.2 Health history

The patient's medical records were used to collect information on the location and type of tumour, age at diagnosis and the main associated comorbidities.

4.2.3 Assessment of nutritional status

Nutritional status was assessed using Standardised Phase Angle analysis through bioimpedance analysis, AGS, anthropometric indicators (percentage weight loss, CB, AMB, DCT) and muscle strength analysis through dynamometry.

4.2.3.1 Electrical Bioimpedance (BIA)

The BIA analysis was carried out using the BIA Quantum X device (RJL systems), which uses a low-intensity current (800 pA) and a frequency of 50 kHz (RJL SYSTEM, 2007). .

Before starting the procedure, the patient was instructed to remove all metal in contact with the skin. The patient was placed in the supine position, with arms and legs separated at a 45° angle. Before placing the electrodes, the contact areas were sanitised with alcohol. The adhesive electrodes were placed in previously standardised locations on the dorsal surface of the foot and hand: a distal electrode at the base of the middle finger and a proximal electrode just above the ankle joint line, between the medial and lateral malleoli and a proximal electrode just above the wrist joint line, coinciding with the styloid process (KYLE *et al.*, 2004a; NORMAN *et al.*, 2010). The resistance, reactance and Phase Angle values were obtained using the *Body Composition* programme, as proposed by the device manufacturer.

The Phase Angle (PA) was calculated in degrees using the formula: tangent arc of the Xc/R ratio already entered into the BIA device; it was then transformed into the standardised phase angle. The Standardised Phase Angle (SFA) was calculated using the equation: SFA = measured PA - mean PA (for age and sex) / population standard deviation for age and sex (PAIVA *et al.*, 2010; BARBOSA-SILVA *et al.*, 2008). Mean PA was obtained using the reference values for sex and age, as proposed by Barbosa-Silva *et al.* (2005a) (TABLE 1). Next, PA values were categorised as being at risk when they were below -1.65 (the cut-off point representing the 5th percentile) and considered to be the lower limit for the healthy population, or not at risk when the values were above -1.65.

TABLE 1 - Phase angle reference values according to age and gender.

| Age (years) | Phase angle | | | |
| | Male | | Female | |
	Average	Standard deviation	Average	Standard deviation
18 - 20	7,90	0,47	7,04	0,85
20 - 29	8,02	0,75	6,98	0,92
30 - 39	8,01	0,85	6,87	0,84
40 - 49	7,76	0,85	6,91	0,85
50 - 59	7,31	0,89	6,55	0,87
60 - 69	6,96	1,10	5,97	0,83
> 70	6,19	0,97	5,64	1,02

Source: Barbosa-Silva *et al.* (2005a).

4.2.3.2 Subjective Global Assessment (SGA)

The SGA was only carried out preoperatively, according to the method proposed by Detsky *et al.* (1987), taking into account the patient's previous weight history and food intake, the metabolic demands of the disease and the physical examination. Subsequently, the final classification of the individual into well-nourished, suspected malnourished/moderately malnourished or severely malnourished was determined. The results of the nutritional status were grouped in order to contemplate the analyses of interest in a dichotomised way into nourished (when the patient's classification was well nourished) and malnourished (when the patient's classification was suspected malnutrition/moderately malnourished and severely malnourished).

4.2.3.3 Anthropometric assessment

Weight was measured using a Tanita Solar Scale® portable digital scale, which has a maximum capacity of 150 kilograms. The patient was instructed to wear as little clothing as possible and to be barefoot. They were positioned in the centre of the equipment, upright, with their feet together and arms extended along their body (BRASIL, 2004).

The percentage of weight loss was calculated according to the following equation: %PPP = patient's usual weight (over the last six months) - current weight / usual weight X 100. This variable was dichotomised, and significant and severe weight loss was considered to be that equal to or greater than 10% of the weight change, and below this percentage was characterised as absence of severe weight loss (BLACKBURN; BISTRIAN, 1977).

Brachial circumference (BC) was measured using an inelastic tape measure with a resolution of 0.1 centimetre (cm) and triceps skinfold (TSF) using a Lange® adipometer, with constant pressure of 10g/mm^2 on the contact surface, precision of 1mm and a scale of 0-65mm. The patient was instructed to flex their right forearm 90° towards their chest and, using a tape measure, the measurement was taken between the tip of the acromial process and the olecranon process in order to obtain the midpoint of the arm length. WC and TCD were measured at the midpoint, with the arm relaxed and extended along the body. TCD was measured at the back of the arm, with the adipometer positioned

perpendicular to the skinfold. For better classification criteria, the value recorded was the average of three consecutive measurements.

Based on these measurements, the arm muscle area (AMB) was calculated using the formulae proposed by Heymsfield et al. (1982). The DCT, CB and AMB results were categorised according to age and gender using the percentiles proposed by Frisancho (1990). Subsequently, the values were dichotomised into nutritional deficit when classified below the fifth percentile, while the others were classified as having no nutritional deficit.

4.2.3.4 Muscle strength assessment

Muscle strength was measured using a Jamar Plus+® dynamometer. During the assessment, the participants were instructed to remain seated on a bench or adjustable bed according to height, with the shoulder in a neutral position, the elbows preferably at 90° and the wrist in a neutral position (intermediate between pronation and supination) with the arm supported (JAMAR, 2000).

Three measurements were taken on the patient's dominant hand, with each contraction lasting three seconds and a rest period of one minute between each one. The average value of the measurements was used. The values obtained were categorised according to age and gender. Values below the fifth percentile (P5) were classified as muscle strength depletion according to Budziareck, Duarte and Barbosa-Silva (2008). The reference values for dynamometry classification used in this study are shown in Table 2.

TABLE 2 - Reference values for dynamometry (Kg) according to gender and age, for the dominant hand.

AGE	MAN		WOMAN	
	P5	**P95**	**P5**	**P95**
18-30 years	30	57	16	30
31-59 years	27	55	16	35
> 60 years	18	44	11	29

Source: Budziareck, Duarte and Barbosa-Silva (2008).

4.2.4 Clinical outcomes

4.2.4.1 Infectious and non-infectious complications

The infectious and non-infectious complications that occurred in the post-operative period were collected daily from the patient's medical records and through reports at bedside. The possible complications described by the *American College of Surgeons* (2000) are listed in Table 1. The following were considered infectious complications: wound infection, pneumonia, bacteraemia, urinary tract infection and sepsis. Non-infectious complications were: fistula, surgical wound dehiscence, haemorrhage, respiratory tract failure, cardiocirculatory failure and renal failure.

TABLE 1 - Definitions of the different types of complications possibly seen in post-operative patients

Complications	Definitions
Pneumonia	Clinical signs or positive culture of tracheal aspirate, blood and/or radiographic evidence
Urinary tract infection	Clinical symptoms or bacteraemia (>100,000 colony forming units/mL)
Bacteraemia	Positive blood culture
Sepsis	Suspected or confirmed infection and fever >38°C or hypotension (systolic pressure < 90mmHg) or oliguria (< 20 mL/h)
Surgical wound dehiscence	Opening > 3cm
Haemorrhage	Need for blood transfusion (> 2IU)
Respiratory tract insufficiency	Presence of dyspnoea and respiratory rate >35 breaths per minute
Cardiocirculatory insufficiency	Unstable blood pressure requiring the administration of fluids or inotropic drugs
Kidney failure	Need for haemodialysis
Fistula	Dehiscence of anastomoses

Source: American College of Surgeons (2000).

4.2.4.2 Hyperglycaemia - Capillary blood glucose

Blood glucose was obtained by recording it in the medical records or, when this information was not available, blood was taken by inserting a drop of capillary blood into a disposable biosensor strip attached to the glucometer (*NICE-SUGAR STUDY INVESTIGATORS et al.*, 2009) by the nursing team or the researcher. The measurements were taken after calibrating the monitor according to the manufacturer's specifications. The test was carried out in accordance with the guidelines in the AccuChek Active® device manufacturer's user manual and the hygiene and asepsis precautions proposed by the SBD guidelines (SOCIEDADE BRASILEIRA DE DIABETES, 2014). Blood glucose was collected at two different times, pre-defined according to the routine of the Alfa Institute of Gastroenterology at the UFMG Hospital das Clínicas: at 6am and 6pm (equivalent to one preprandial and one postprandial capillary blood glucose collection), using the average obtained from these values.

The results obtained were classified according to the criteria proposed by the *American Diabetes Association* (ADA, 2010), which considers a limit of 140mg/dL to be hyperglycaemia in a hospital environment.

4.2.4.3 Length of hospital stay

The length of hospital stay was obtained by calculating the number of days between the date of admission and discharge. The values were also categorised according to the length of stay described in the literature (>16 days) (BAPEN., 2003; RASLAN *et al.*, 2010) and presented by median.

4.2.4.4 Mortality rate

The occurrence of death was assessed during the patients' hospitalisation, by means of a survey of the medical records or during weekly bed checks at the Alfa Institute of Medicine.
Gastroenterology, and the mortality rate is calculated from this data.

4.3 . Data processing and analysis

The data was analysed using the *Statistical Package for the Social Sciences for Windows Student Version®* (SPSS), version 20.0. The variables were descriptively analysed by calculating frequency distributions and measures of central tendency and dispersion. Variables with a normal distribution, verified using the Kolmogorov-Smirnov test, were presented as means (standard deviation) while the others were presented as medians (25th-75th percentile-p_{75}).

To check the association of nutritional status variables with gender, age and tumour site, Student's t-test and Fisher's chi-square/exact test were used to compare independent means and proportions, respectively. The Anova test for repeated measures and McNemar's test were applied to compare the means and proportions of the variables relating to nutritional status and glycaemic control at the preoperative stage, using Bonferroni as a *post-hoc* test.

The association of AFP with anthropometric indicators and clinical outcomes was assessed using logistic regression, with categorised AFP used as the explanatory variable in all models. In the logistic regression models, the dependent variables were anthropometric indicators and clinical outcomes in dichotomised form, and in these models the *odds ratio* (*OR*) was used as the measure of effect, with a 95% confidence interval (95% CI). All the models were also adjusted for possible confounding factors (tumour location and length of hospital stay). The model for predicting capillary glycaemia was also adjusted for the presence of diabetes.

The agreement between the diagnosis of malnutrition was assessed preoperatively using the AFP and the nutritional status assessment criteria commonly used in the Alfa Institute's practice: AGS, dynanometry and AMB. This was done by calculating the kappa value between pairs of the different definitions. The degree of agreement between the definitions of malnutrition was assessed according to the following kappa value categories: a) < 0.20 = very poor; b) 0.21 to 0.40 = poor; c) 0.41 to 0.60 = moderate; d) 0.61 to 0.80 = good; e) > 0.80 = very good (LANDIS; KOCH, 1977).

To compare the capillary glycaemia means between patients with and without nutritional risk, according to the AFP categorisation, the Ancova test was carried out, adjusted for the presence of diabetes. It should be noted that this study presented the adjusted means generated by this analysis. The Mann-Whitney test was used to compare the medians of hospitalisation time according to the AFP classification. Finally, Cox regression was used, with death as the dependent variable and dichotomised AFP as the explanatory variable. This model was adjusted for tumour site. The significant association between the variables was calculated using the Hazard Ratio (HR), which took into account the length of hospitalisation of each patient.

The significance level adopted for all statistical analyses was 5% (p<0.05).

CHAPTER 5

RESULTS

5.1 Characterisation of the sample

5.1.1 General characterisation

Between September 2014 and October 2015, 164 hospitalised cancer patients were eligible for this study. Of these, 28 did not have their data collected at the time of assessment and 15 patients had their operation cancelled or postponed, making a total of 121 patients included in the study.

The average age of the patients was 58.8 ±12.5 years, and the highest prevalence (52.9%) was male. With regard to the main associated comorbidities, 62% and 20% of patients had hypertension and diabetes, respectively. The average time since cancer diagnosis was 10 ±14.5 months and patients with colon and rectal tumours accounted for 47.9% of the cases.

The nutritional status of the patients in the preoperative period, according to the different nutritional status indicators used at the Alfa Institute, is shown in Table 3. It was observed that 28.1% of the patients were at nutritional risk, according to the AFP classification, and that the prevalence of malnutrition, according to the AGS, was 63.6%. It was found that 45% and 27% of patients were nutritionally deficient according to the arm circumference (AC) and triceps skinfold (TSF) classifications, respectively. More than half of the patients (53.2%) had AMB values below the fifth percentile and 16.5% had muscle strength depletion assessed by dynamometry (TABLE 3).

TABLE 3 - General characteristics and preoperative nutritional status of surgical oncology patients.

Variables	Total	
	N	%
Sex		
Male	64	52,9
Age group		
30-39 years	10	8,3
40-49 years old	16	13,2
50-59 years	42	34,7
60-69 years	26	21,5
>70 years	27	22,3
Tumour location		
EED	33	27,3
CCP	15	12,4
COLOP	58	47,9
FVB	15	12,4

Standardised Phase Angle		
At Risk (<-1.65)	34	28,1
Subjective Global Assessment		
Malnourished	76	63,6
Arm circumference		
Nutritional Deficit	54	45,0
Tricipital skinfold		
Nutritional Deficit	33	27,0
Arm Muscle Area		
Nutritional Deficit	64	53,2
Dynamometry		
Muscle Strength Depletion	20	16,5

Acronyms: EED (stomach, intestine and duodenum); CCP (head and neck); COLOP (colon and rectum); FVB (liver and bile ducts).
Source: Research data. Alfa Institute of Gastroenterology/HC/UFMG (n=121), Belo Horizonte, 2016.

5.2 Association between nutritional status depletion and tumour location

The results of the association between preoperative nutritional status measured by different indicators and AFP, according to tumour location, are shown in Table 4. The highest prevalence of nutritional risk was observed, according to the AFP classification, among patients with FVB cancer (66.7%), compared to those diagnosed with EED cancer (24.3%), CCP (13.4%) and COLOP (24.1%); (p=0.004). Patients with FVB tumours (73.3%) were also more malnourished according to different parameters, such as the CB classification (p=0.001), compared to patients with colon and rectum tumours (28.1%), and had a higher percentage of muscle strength depletion (42.9%) compared to patients with head and neck tumours (0.0%). There was no statistical difference between groups when assessing AMB.

TABLE 4 - Depletion of nutritional status diagnosed by different methods, according to the location of the tumour in surgical oncology patients.

Variable	Tumour site (%)				p-value*
	EED (N=33)	CCP (N=15)	COLOP (N=58)	FVB (N=15)	
Standardised Phase Angle With Risk	24,3[a]	13,4[a]	24,1[a]	66,7[b]	**0,004**
Subjective Global Assessment Malnourished	60,6	60,0	67,2	60,0	0,890
Arm Circumference With Nutritional Deficit	63,6[a]	40,0[ab]	28,1[b]	73,3[a]	**0,001**
Tricipital skinfold with nutritional deficit	32,3	40,0	20,0	26,7	0,397
Nutritionally Deficient Arm Muscle Area	67,7[a]	40,0[a]	42,0[a]	73,3[a]	**0,034**
Dynamometry Depletion of Muscle Strength	12,1[ab]	0,0[a]	13,8[ab]	42,9[b]	**0,001**

Abbreviations: EED (stomach, intestine and duodenum); CCP (head and neck); COLOP (colon and rectum); FVB (liver and bile ducts). Values expressed as a percentage.
*Chi-Square/Fisher's Exact test for comparing proportions. Percentage values with common letters on the same line are statistically equal and statistical significance is established by the Bonferroni correction (p>0.0083).
Source: Research data. Alfa Institute of Gastroenterology/HC/UFMG (n=121), Belo Horizonte, 2016.

In this study, when comparing the mean age between malnourished and well-nourished patients according to the different nutritional indicators assessed, no significant difference was observed (p>0.05). With regard to gender, a significant difference was found in men according to the CB classification (57.8 per cent *vs.* 30.4 per cent, p= 0.003) and AMB (72.6 per cent *vs.* 28.6 per cent, p< 0.001), compared to women, with no difference for the other indicators (p<0.05).

5.3 Association between AFP and preoperative nutritional indicators

The association between AFP and nutritional status indicators is shown in Table 5:

TABLE 5 - Simple logistic regression models for associations between being at nutritional risk according to the AFP classification and indicators of nutritional status, preoperatively.

Dependent variables	With risk for AFP (OR; 95% CI)	p-value*
Subjective Global Assessment Nourished Malnourished	1 3,66 (1,35-9,90)	**0,010**
Dynamometry Normal Muscle Strength Muscle Strength Depletion	1 3,84 (1,31-11,25)	**0,011**
Arm circumference Normal or Increased Mass Deficit	1 4,24 (1,72-10,43)	**0,002**
Arm Muscle Area Normal or High Low or Below Average	1 4,38 (1,68-11,42)	**0,002**
Triceps skinfold No Deficit Severe or Mild Deficit	1 1,86 (0,74-4,69)	0,184
Body weight loss < 10% > 10%	1 3,86 (1,64-9,06)	**0,002**

1Regression model adjusted by tumour site. The explanatory variable in each regression model was the AFP variable (0 >without nutritional risk and 1 >with nutritional risk). Note: CI = confidence interval; OR = Odds Ratio.
Source: Research data. Alfa Institute of Gastroenterology/HC/UFMG (n=121), Belo Horizonte, 2016.

A simple logistic regression model was carried out for each anthropometric indicator in its dichotomised form (AGS, dynamometry, CB, AMB, DCT and PPP), adjusted by tumour site and with AFP as the explanatory variable. It was observed that, preoperatively, individuals at nutritional risk according to the AFP categorisation were more likely to be malnourished, according to AGS (OR=3.66; 95% CI: 1.35-9.90), CB (OR=4.24; 95% CI: 1.72-10.43), AMB (OR=4.38; 95% CI: 1.68-11.42), and to have a higher percentage of severe weight loss (PPP) (OR=3.86; 95% CI: 1.64-9.06). With regard to dynamometry, it was observed that patients classified as being at risk by the

AFP were 3.84 (95% CI: 1.31-11.25) times more likely to have muscle strength depletion (p<0.05).

5.4 Analysis of agreement between AFP and nutritional indicators

The agreement between being at risk according to the AFP classification and the nutritional status indicators used at the Alfa Institute of Gastroenterology (AGS, dynamometry and AMB) is shown in Table 6. It can be seen that there was significant but weak agreement between the AFP and all the indicators assessed preoperatively (p<0.05).

TABLE 6 - Concordance between being at risk according to the AFP classification and different indicators of nutritional status, preoperatively.

Reference method	Total (N=121) (*kappa coefficient/* p-value)
Subjective Global Assessment	0,29 (p=0,001)
Arm Muscle Area	0,24 (p=0,003)
Dynamometry	0,25 (p=0,003)

Source: Research data. Alfa Institute of Gastroenterology/HC/UFMG (n=121), Belo Horizonte, 2016.

5.5 Characterisation and association between AFP, glycaemia and clinical outcomes

In this study, a high prevalence of infectious complications (57.0%) was identified among the oncology patients assessed. Patients classified as being at risk according to the AFP classification were 3.51 (95% CI: 1.37-8.99; p=0.009) times more likely to have infectious complications during their hospital stay. There was no association between the AFP and the other outcomes assessed (p>0.05) (TABLE 7).

TABLE 7 - Logistic regression analysis for associations between AFP and clinical outcomes in the preoperative period

Dependent variables	Preoperative AFP (OR; 95% CI)	p-value*
Infectious complications No Yes		
	1	
	3,51 (1,37-8,99)	**0,009**
Non-Infectious Complications No		
Yes	1	
	1,25 (0,51-3,02)	0,619
Preoperative glycaemia		
Normoglycaemia < 140mg/dL Hospital	1	
hyperglycaemia > 140mg/dL	0,43 (0,06-2,77)	0,378
Length of Hospital Stay < 16 days > 16		
days	1	
	0,348 (0,04-3,02)	0,348

*Regression models adjusted for tumour site and length of stay. In the case of capillary glycaemia, also adjusted for the presence of diabetes. The explanatory variable in each regression model was AFP (0 >without

nutritional risk and 1 >with nutritional risk). Note: CI = confidence interval; OR = Odds Ratio.
Source: Research data. Alfa Institute of Gastroenterology/HC/UFMG (n=121), Belo Horizonte, 2016.

The frequency of patients who went to the intensive care unit (ICU) represented 36.4% of the sample (N=44). The median length of ICU stay was 0 (0-5) and the median length of hospital stay was 6 (5-9) days. The mortality rate found during the patients' stay was 3.3%, totalling 4 deaths.

With regard to capillary glycaemia assessment in the sub-sample collected (n=50), it was observed that 33.3% of the patients had in-hospital hyperglycaemia in the post-operative period. The average glycaemic levels were 120±33 mg/dL, 135 ±37 mg/dL and 125 ±37 mg/dL at the preoperative, postoperative and hospital discharge times, respectively. In the paired analysis, it was found that the mean glycaemia at the post-operative moment was higher than at hospital discharge (p<0.05). However, there was no significant difference in glycaemia between the pre- and post-operative periods (p>0.05) and between the pre-operative period and hospital discharge (p>0.05). On the other hand, the data obtained when comparing the mean blood glucose levels using the ancova test, adjusted for the presence of diabetes, indicates that there was a difference with a significant trend, according to the AFP categorisation, only at the preoperative stage, with those patients classified as being at nutritional risk, according to the AFP categorisation, having a higher mean blood glucose level than those patients classified as being at no risk (133.11±8.7 vs. 115.99±4.6, p=0.089).

When comparing the length of hospital stay, it was observed that there was no significant difference in the length of hospital stay between those patients identified as being at risk by the AFP (median: 6.00, p25: 5.00, p75: 9.00) compared to those characterised as being not at risk (median: 7.00, p25: 5.00, p75: 9.25) according to the AFP categorisation (p=0.720). It was also observed that there was no significant difference in the risk of death rate between those patients classified as at risk or not at risk, according to the AFP categorisation (HR: 2.37; 95% CI: 0.33-16.88, p=0.387).

CHAPTER 6

DISCUSSION

The use of Phase Angle as a predictor of body cell mass and, consequently, a possible marker of nutritional status, and to predict clinical outcomes and survival, has been evaluated over the last decade (BARBOSA- SILVA, 2005; PAIVA *et al.*, 2010; KYLE et *al.*, 2012; NORMAN *et al.*, 2012; MALECKA-MASSALSKA *et al.*, 2015).

However, there are still controversies about this indicator, since most studies have used PA in degrees and in patients with different types of illnesses, which makes it difficult to use and interpret, since PA can vary according to different determinants such as: underlying disease, population, gender and age (SUITA; YAMANOUCHI, 2000; BARBOSA-SILVA *et al*, 2005a; BOSY-WESTPHAL *et al.*, 2006; BARBOSA-SILVA *et al.*, 2008; NORMAN *et al.*, 2010; SCHEUNEMANN *et al.*, 2011).

In this study, it is important to note that we chose to use the Standardised Phase Angle (SPA) instead of the Phase Angle in degrees. This choice was due to the fact that the Phase Angle in degrees can be altered according to gender and age, as well as varying depending on the study population (BARBOSA-SILVA *et al.*, 2008; PAIVA *et al.*, 2010; NORMAN et *al.*, 2012). As the AFP is a value adjusted for age, gender and takes into account the standard deviation (SD), values lower than the fifth percentile for the healthy population (BARBOSA- SILVA, 2005) could be more effective in indicating changes in patients' state of health than absolute values, given in degrees (BARBOSA-SILVA 2008; NORMAN *et al.*, 2010; PAIVA *et al.*, *2010*). In this sense, the main hypothesis of this study was to investigate whether AFP could be used as a method of assessing nutritional status in hospitalised cancer patients, as well as to check its relationship with hospital hyperglycaemia and whether it could be a potential predictor of adverse clinical outcomes.

The patients' nutritional status was assessed using different parameters. A high prevalence (63.6%) of malnourished patients was found preoperatively, according to the AGS classification. In relation to dynamometry, 16.5% of patients showed signs of muscle strength depletion, while the classification of nutritional status assessed using the BC and AMB showed that more than half of the patients studied had nutritional deficits. These prevalences are higher than those described in the literature. In a recent study, Barbosa-Silva *et al.* (2014) assessed 66 patients diagnosed with colorectal cancer and found that 36.4% of the patients were malnourished according to the AGS. In another recent study, Fernandez *et al.* (2014) assessed the nutritional status of 201 patients admitted to a university hospital and reported that 11.9% were classified as malnourished using the AGS, with the highest prevalence of malnutrition being detected in patients admitted to the oncology and haematology department. In the study by Malecka-Massalska *et al.* (2015) on 75 patients with head and neck cancer, 40% of the individuals were found to be malnourished according to the AGS classification (32% were diagnosed with moderate malnutrition and 8% with severe malnutrition). This data confirms that the prevalence of malnutrition in the hospital environment is still high.

With regard to AFP, 28.1% of patients had low values (<5th percentile; <-1.65) preoperatively. This prevalence was similar to that found in the study by Paixão *et al.* (2015) in which 104 hospitalised radiotherapy patients were assessed and 27% of patients were found to be below the fifth percentile (<-1.65), according to the AFP classification for the Brazilian population. In a study by the group of Cardinal *et al.* (2010), carried out on 125 patients who were also hospitalised in the preoperative period, it was observed that 20% of the patients were below the 5th percentile for a healthy population; however, using a cut-off point of (< - 0.8). In contrast to these findings, Norman *et al.* (2010) reported a much higher prevalence in a study of 399 cancer patients, with 78% of patients classified as having AFP below the fifth percentile. It is speculated that this difference may be explained by the reference value used by this group, which was for the German population, differing from the cut-off point in the present study.

The high prevalence of malnutrition found in this study can be explained by the low socio-economic and cultural conditions of these patients, most of whom have late and restricted access to public medical services. In addition, patients diagnosed with cancer in different locations (head and neck, colon and rectum, liver and biliary tract) were included. It is known that the location of the tumour is an important factor that has a significant impact on the patient's nutritional status and may also be one of the factors related to the high prevalence of malnutrition found in this study.

The association between tumour location and nutritional status was assessed. It was observed that patients with BFV tumours were more malnourished in terms of different parameters compared to other tumour sites according to the AFP classification, as well as having a higher percentage of muscle strength depletion compared to patients diagnosed with head and neck cancer. According to Jensen *et al.* (2009), patients with hepatocarcinoma have an increased risk of malnutrition, since the liver is the central organ of metabolism and is directly involved in various reactions, especially those involving macro and micronutrients. In addition, hepatocellular carcinoma is more difficult to stage than other solid tumours because most patients with this diagnosis have underlying liver dysfunction, as well as an exacerbated tumour burden (HOFF *et al.*, 2013; THOMAS, 2013). Nevertheless, around 20 to 30% of liver tumours, especially those smaller than 10 mm, are not easily identified with any technique, leading to late diagnosis with advanced stages of the disease (LLOVET *et al.*, 2003; MALFERTHEINER, 2015). Thus, delays in both diagnosis and treatment can trigger negative repercussions that impact on the nutritional status of these patients (JENSEN *et al.*, 2009; LLOVET *et al.*, 2003; BOZZETTI *et al.*, 2012).

Other factors related to nutritional status are gender and age. In this study, when comparing the mean age between malnourished and well-nourished patients, according to the different nutritional indicators assessed, there was no significant difference (p>0.05). With regard to gender, a significant difference was found between men, according to the CB classification (57.8 per cent *vs.* 30.4 per cent, p= 0.003) and AMB (72.6 per cent *vs.* 28.6 per cent, p< 0.001), compared to women, with no difference for the other indicators. A similar result was found by Cardinal *et al.* (2010) in a study of 125 surgical patients. The authors observed greater nutritional depletion, according to the AMB classification, among men when compared to women (46.6 per cent *vs.* 16.4 per cent). According to Schraiber *et al.* (2010), males seek health services later, when they usually already have the disease or are in more advanced stages of the pathology, thus impacting on their nutritional status.

As for age, our results differ from those described in the literature. Azevedo *et al.* (2006) in a study of 136 hospitalised patients found that age was related to malnutrition. According to Kyle *et al.* (2012), elderly individuals find it more difficult to recover their nutritional status due to the metabolic and physiological changes resulting from the ageing process itself. Pirlich *et al.* (2005) found that patients aged 80 or over were five times more likely to be malnourished than those under 50. In this study, the average age was 58±12.5 years. It is therefore believed that the fact that the patients under study were not of advanced age may have been one of the reasons why no associations were found with nutritional status.

A simple logistic regression model was used to analyse the association between AFP and preoperative nutritional status indicators. This showed that individuals at nutritional risk, according to the AFP categorisation, were more likely to be malnourished, according to AGS, CB, AMB, and to have a higher PPP. With regard to dynamometry, it was observed that patients categorised as being at risk by the AFP were also more likely to have muscle strength depletion (p<0.05). These results are in line with the relationship between PA and body cell mass. Thus, changes in MCC due to altered nutritional status can result in changes in PA (BARBOSA-SILVA *et al.*, 2003). In addition, functional impairment is directly associated with muscle strength depletion, reflecting a decrease in lean body mass (MONTANO-LOZA *et al.*, 2015; SCHUTTE; SCHULZ; MALFERTHEINER, 2015), which could also interfere with AFP values.

With regard to dynamometry, the study by Norman *et al.* (2009) assessed 189 patients with different types of cancer and showed that dynamometry values were significantly lower in patients diagnosed with malnutrition by AGS when compared to well-nourished patients. The authors concluded that malnutrition is an independent risk factor for reduced muscle strength in this population. According to Barbosa-Silva *et al.* (2008), changes in functionality assessed using dynamometry would be observed prior to changes in anthropometric parameters such as AMB, CB, DCT in the presence of malnutrition. In this way, it can be inferred that cellular and functional markers change earlier in the presence of changes in the nutritional status of hospitalised patients, making it useful for assessment in a hospital environment. The relationship between AFP and dynamometry was also evaluated by Norman *et al.* (2010). The authors studied 399 oncological patients and showed that AFP was considered a good predictor for identifying altered functional status, as measured by muscle strength. In a study evaluating patients with colon and rectal cancer, it was observed that an increase in PA was associated with an increase in the physical function scale and a reduction in fatigue, demonstrating an improvement in the functional aspects and quality of life of these patients (GUPTA *et al.*, 2009). It is known that muscle strength is reduced, especially in cancer patients, since the catabolism in which these patients find themselves can directly affect skeletal muscle fibres, with a consequent reduction in muscle strength, thus interfering in the functionality of these individuals (NORMAN *et al.*, 2011; LIMBERGER *et al.*, 2014).

Few studies have evaluated AFP with other markers of nutritional status such as CB and AMB in surgical patients. In the study carried out by Cardinal *et al.* (2010) with 125 hospitalised surgical patients in the preoperative phase, a lower mean AFP value was observed in malnourished patients, according to AMB (kappa=0.20). In the study by Peres *et al.* (2012) of 66 patients admitted to a university hospital, higher PA values, measured in degrees, were positively correlated with anthropometric measurements of WC (r = 0.29, p = 0.015) and BMA (r = 0.29, p = 0.023).

In the present study, AFP was also associated with the percentage of weight loss, and being at risk according to the AFP categorisation increased the chances of the patient having a percentage of severe weight loss (>10%) by 3.86 times. It is known that involuntary weight loss is present in almost 85% of patients with different types of tumour (PAIVA *et al.*, 2010). Although not used in isolation in nutritional assessment, evidence suggests that weight loss of more than 5% of the patient's usual weight in the last six months is associated with reduced food intake and systemic inflammation. This can be indicative of cachexia and can lead to progressive metabolic abnormalities, electrolyte disturbances and immunological deficits, which are also associated with increased complications and mortality (MARIN CARO *et al.*, 2008; GONZALEZ-SILVIA *et al.*, 2013). Similar results were found in a recent study by Paixão, Gonzalez and Ito (2015) on 104 cancer patients undergoing radiotherapy, in which a 1 kg reduction in body weight corresponded to a 0.107 degree reduction in PA ($p<0.0001$).

In the present study, preoperative AFP was also associated with SGA. Individuals at risk according to the AFP classification were approximately four times more likely to be malnourished according to the SGA classification. This result is in line with that found by Scheunemann *et al.* (2011) in a study of 98 patients admitted for gastrointestinal surgery. These authors showed that patients diagnosed as malnourished by AGS had significantly lower AFP compared to the average of those who were well-nourished. Another study of hospitalised patients with gastrointestinal disease showed that there was a gradual decrease in Phase Angle according to the classification of malnutrition by AGS (NORMAN *et al.*, 2008). The study by Barbosa-Silva (2005a) also showed that the Phase Angle was closely related to the nutritional status of hospitalised patients, according to the SGA, at the preoperative stage.

The kappa test was carried out to assess whether the AFP had good agreement with the different methods of identifying nutritional status (AGS, AMB and dynamometry) used in the practice of the Alfa Institute of Gastroenterology. It was observed that, preoperatively, there was significant ($p<0.05$) but weak agreement between the AFP and all the reference methods for assessing nutritional status (AGS, k=0.29; AMB, k=0.24; Dynamometry, k=0.25). The kappa coefficient values found in this study were close to the coefficients reported by Scheunemann *et al.* (2011) who assessed pre-surgical patients, 15% of whom had gastrointestinal cancer, and found low agreement between PA and AGS (kappa=0.27), and among patients with colon and rectal cancer, Gupta *et al.* (2008) found kappa=0.33. In the study by Barbosa-Silva *et al.* (2003) which assessed 279 hospitalised patients in the preoperative period, lower PA values (PA < 5th percentile) were observed in patients classified as malnourished using the SGA, with better agreement (kappa=0.39), but agreement was also considered poor. According to Scheunemann *et al.* (2011), the low level of agreement found between PFA and other methods of assessing nutritional status may be due to the fact that PA and nutritional status indicators express different aspects and levels of nutritional deficiency. Barbosa-Silva *et al.* (2008) stated that the first stage to be altered during the malnutrition process is related to molecular alterations, such as changes in cell membranes, which can be observed using the Phase Angle.

In this sense, because it is capable of reflecting molecular alterations, AFP would be an earlier indicator than anthropometry, for example, in detecting malnutrition (BARBOSA-SILVA *et al.*, 2008). However, more studies are needed to confirm the use of PA as a nutritional assessment and monitoring method, since the findings of this study suggest that AFP cannot be used as a reference assessment method, since it did not show good agreement with the methods used in the hospital environment.

With regard to clinical outcomes, it was observed that the prevalence of infectious complications was present in more than half of the study sample (57.0%) and that these were associated with PFA (p<0.05). Phase Angle is known to be based on reactance measurements, which in turn are associated with mass function and cell membrane integrity. These may be compromised by the release of inflammatory cytokines, derived from the presence of the tumour itself, and by altered homeostasis in cancer surgical patients. In this way, these individuals would be at greater risk of complications, especially infectious ones (HUI *et al.*, 2014). Barbosa Silva *et al.* (2005a) also observed that patients with lower Phase Angle values were more prone to high risks of complications after surgical procedures.

It should be noted that few studies have assessed the potential of AFP to predict complications, whether infectious or non-infectious (SCHWENK *et al.*, 2000; BARBOSA-SILVA, 2005a; HUI *et al.*, 2014). Most authors have evaluated and related PA to survival (TOSO *et al.*, 2000; SELBERG; SELBERG, 2002; GUPTA et *al.* 2004a; AZEVEDO et *al.*, 2006; GUPTA et *al.*, 2008; HUI et *al.*, 2009; SONSIN et *al.*, 2009; PAIVA et al., 2010; NORMAN *et al., 2010;* LLAMES et al., 2013; HUI *et al.*, 2014). Gupta *et al.* (2004a) and Gupta *et al.*

(2004b), evaluating patients with pancreatic and colorectal cancer, showed that PA values lower than 5 degrees were related to a worse prognosis and also to a shorter survival time than patients evaluated with higher PA. According to Hui *et al.* (2014), who assessed 222 patients diagnosed with advanced cancer, those classified with an AFP lower than the fifth percentile had an increased risk of post-surgical complications. Barbosa-Silva *et al.* (2005b) compared PA with other nutritional parameters and also with prognostic factors for post-surgical complications. The authors showed that, even after analysis adjusted for gender and age, PA also remained associated with a worse prognosis. These results indicate that PA, as well as being a marker of cellular function, can be a predictive factor of the risk of adverse complications and survival.

The concept of stress-induced hyperglycaemia is not new and interest in the subject has been growing since Van Den Berghe (2001) showed that strict control of glycaemia (80-110mg/dL) with continuous intravenous insulin was associated with lower morbidity (sepsis, blood transfusion) and mortality in hospitalised patients (it should be noted that 60% of the population in this study was made up of post-operative patients). This study found that 33.3% of patients had hyperglycaemia in hospital (blood glucose >140mg\dL), with a significant mean difference between the post-operative period and hospital discharge (p<0.05). These results were to be expected, given that in the post-operative period, patients undergoing surgery show various metabolic changes due to the systemic response to the surgical trauma, with the main purpose of providing cellular fuel at a time of increased metabolic demand, a frequent phenomenon in the hospital environment (WAITZBERG *et al.*, 2001; LEITE *et al.*, 2010; BONAMICHI et *al.*, 2015). Furthermore, most of the patients were assessed close to the peak of the inflammatory response, i.e. on the third postoperative day (3rd PO day), when there is also a peak in the concentration of pro-inflammatory cytokines, mainly IL-6, IL-1 and TNFa, with a concomitant increase in the production of counter-regulatory hormones such as cortisol, glucagon and catecholamines, with an increase in peripheral resistance to insulin action and an increase in total energy expenditure (WAITZBERG *et al.*, 2001; BRIASSOULIS *et al.*, 2009; WEIMANN *et al.*, 2009). These changes can lead to different disorders, such as cellular glycotoxicity (LEITE *et al.*, 2010;
BONAMICHI *et al.*, 2015; SOCIEDADE BRASILEIRA DE DIABETES, 2015b) and could directly affect the health of the membranes, thus possibly interfering with the PA of these patients. However, capillary glycaemia was not associated with PA in our study (p>0.05). For these results, it could be speculated that the fact that blood was collected capillary may have caused interference in relation to venous collection, since the margin of error between the forms measured can vary between 20% and 25% (SACKS *et al.*, 2003). It is also believed that the extreme deleterious effect of glucocorticoid with an impact on the cell membrane occurs at even higher blood glucose values than those observed, when there is no bolus correction and adequate treatment in the hospital routine; which was not the practice in our service (ACE/ADA, 2009; BRAZILIAN DIABETES SOCIETY, 2015a). However, no other studies were found that had assessed this situation. The data obtained from the comparison of mean blood glucose levels indicates that patients

classified as being at risk according to the AFP had higher mean blood glucose levels than patients classified as not being at risk (133.11 ±8.7 vs. 115.99±4.6, p=0.089) in the preoperative period. It is believed that these results may have been influenced mainly by the fact that glycaemia collection took place in a sub-sample (N=50) due to the difficulty of collection, a period of financial adjustments, a hospital strike, among other factors inherent to the Institute's routine, thus impacting on the sample power (30%) assessed. However, no studies have been found to date that have assessed this association. These are plausible findings and suggest that further studies are needed in order to verify and deepen the possible association between AFP and hyperglycaemia (regardless of the patient's previous diagnosis of diabetes), since this is so common in the hospital environment; as well as future studies that could assess the impact of glycaemic changes on adverse outcomes in surgical oncology patients.

Non-infectious complications, length of ICU stay and death, were not associated with AFP in this study, although it is known that the worse the patient's nutritional status, the longer the hospital stay, the greater the vulnerability to readmissions, increased complications and infections (WAITZBERG *et al.*, 2001; HUMMAN MB *et al., 2005;* JOSEP-ARGILÉS *et al.,* 2014), it is believed that the short average period of hospitalisation and evaluation to which the patients were subjected. in this study, may have contributed to these results. Fernandez *et al.* (2014) also found no association between PFA, length of stay and death during hospitalisation of hospitalised patients (p>0.05).

It should be emphasised that this study has some limitations. Tumour staging was not assessed in relation to the variables of interest, which could have influenced the results. It is known that staging is considered an important prognostic tool that provides a classification of tumour severity in order to help guide and plan treatment (HOFF *et al.,* 2013; THOMAS, 2013). Another limitation is that the type of nutritional therapy administered, as well as the water supply and the mortality rate after discharge, were not collected. These could also interfere with the results. Therefore, future studies are needed to demonstrate whether AFP can be modified by the type of nutritional intervention received and whether this would have an impact on a better prognosis in surgical oncology patients.

This work has potential. To our knowledge, this is the first study to investigate whether PA could be used as a diagnostic method for nutritional status in surgical cancer patients. There is also a lack of studies in the literature investigating whether PA is a potential predictor of adverse clinical outcomes and not just survival in these patients.

Furthermore, few studies have compared PA with different parameters commonly used in the hospital environment and, to our knowledge, no study to date has evaluated the supposed association of AFP with hospital hyperglycaemia.

From this perspective, it can be concluded that because AFP is a measure that assesses cellular integrity and makes it possible to evaluate nutritional risk in a more objective way, it could help health professionals in the assessment of nutritional status in hospitalised patients, in order to optimise metabolic assessment, nutritional classification and, consequently, treatment. In the study presented here, PA was associated with AGS, dynamometry and anthropometric parameters commonly used in hospital settings: CB, AMB and weight loss percentage. Therefore, PA can be considered a useful tool to help classify the nutritional status of cancer patients. The findings also suggest that AFP was a good marker and prognostic indicator, capable of predicting infectious complications and showed a significant trend of association in relation to capillary glycaemia in the surgical oncology patients assessed.

Future research is needed to examine the different physiological and cellular changes associated with the Phase Angle, in different populations and in the hospital environment throughout hospitalisation. This could also confirm whether AFP could be used in combination with other diagnostic tools in hospitalised patients, in order to increase sensitivity in detecting impaired nutritional status and its possible relationship with cellular glucotoxicity.

CHAPTER 7

REFERENCES

ACE/ADA. American Association of Clinical Endocrinologists and American Diabetes Association Consensus Statement on Inpatient Glycemic Control. *Endocrine Practice*. v. 15, n. 4, p. 1-17, 2009.

ACUNA, K.; CRUZ, T Evaluation of the nutritional status of adults and the elderly and the nutritional situation of the Brazilian population. *Arq Bras Endocrinol Metab*, São Paulo, v. 48, n.3, p.345-361, Jun. 2004. Available at: <http://www.scielo.br/scielo.php?script=sci_arttext&pid=S0004-27302004000300004&lng=en&nrm=iso>. Accessed on 12 April 2016.

ALLISON, S. P. Malnutrition, disease, and outcome. *Nutrition*. v.16, n.7-8, p.590-593, 2000.

ÁLVAREZ-HERNÁNDEZ, J. *et al*. Prevalence and costs of malnutrition in hospitalised patients; The Predyces Study. *Nutr Hosp*. v. 27, n.4, p.1049-1059, 2012.

ALVES, F.D.; et al. Prognostic role of phase angle in hospitalised patients with acute decompensated heart failure. *Clin Nutr*. pii: S0261-5614(16)30024-3. 2016.

AMERICAN COLLEGE OF SURGEONS. *Bulletin of the American College of Surgeons*. 2000. Available at: <http://bulletin.facs.org/>. Accessed on: 02 Apr. 2016.

ARGILÉS, J.M. *et al*. Physiopathology of neoplastic cachexia. *Nutricion Hospitalaria*, Spain, v. 21, n.3, p. 4-9, 2006.

ASPEN. Board of Directors and the Clinical Guidelines Task Force.Guidelines for the use of parenteral and enteral nutrition in adult and paediatric patients. *JPEN J Parenter Enteral Nutr*. v.26, n.1 Suppl, p.1SA-138SA, 2002.

AZEVEDO, L. C. *et al*. Prevalence of malnutrition in a large general hospital in Santa Catarina/Brazil. *ACM arq. catarin. Med*. v.35. n.4, p.89-96, Oct.-Dec. 2006.

BADIA-TAHULL, M.B. *et al*. Use of Subjective Global Assessment, Patient-Generated Subjective Global Assessment and Nutritional Risk Screening 2002 to evaluate the nutritional status of non-critically ill patients on parenteral nutrition. *Nutr Hosp*. v.29, n.2, p.411-429, 2014.

BALDASSO, E. *et al*. Hyperglycaemia and the use of insulin in critically ill children. *Sci Med*, v.16 , n.2, p.73-78, 2006. Available at: <http://revistaseletronicas.pucrs.br/ojs/index.php/scientiamedica/article/download/162 4/1198>. Accessed on: 05 Apr. 2016.

BARBOSA, L.R.L.S; LACERDA-FILHO, A.; BARBOSA, L.C.L.S. Immediate preoperative nutritional status of patients with colorectal cancer: a warning. *Arq. Gastroenterol*., São Paulo . v. 51, n. 4, p. 331-336, Dec. 2014 .

BARBOSA-SILVA, M. C. *et al*. Reference values for phase angle in the Brazilian population. *Rev Bras Med*. v.65, p.104-105, 2008.

BARBOSA-SILVA, M. C. *et al* Bioelectrical impedance analysis: population reference values for phase angle by age and sex. *Am J Clin Nutr.*, v. 82, n.1, p. 49-52, 2005a.

BARBOSA-SILVA, M. C. *et al.* Can Bioelectrical impedance analysis identify malnutrition in preoperative nutrition assessment. *Nutrition.* v.19, n.5, p.422-426, 2003.

BARBOSA-SILVA, M.C. *et al.* Comparison of phase angle between normal individuals and chemotherapy patients using age and sex reference values. *JPEN J Parenter Enteral Nutr.* v.29, p.S32, 2005b.

BARBOSA-SILVA, M. C.; BARROS, A. J. D. Bioelectrical impedance analysis in clinical practice: a new perspective on its use beyond body composition equations. *Curr Opin Clin Nutr Metab Care.* v.8, n.3, p. 311-317, 2005b.

BARBOSA-SILVA, M.C.; BARROS, A. J. Bioelectric impedance and individual characteristics as prognostic factors for post-operative complications. *Clin Nutr.* v.24, n.5, p.830-848, 2005a.

BARBOSA-SILVA, M.C.G.; BARROS, A.J.D. Subjective nutritional assessment: Part 1 - Review of its validity after two decades of use. *Arq. Gastroenterol.* São Paulo, v.39, n.3, p.181-187, Jul 2002. Available at: <http://www.scielo.br/scielo.php?pid=S0004-28032002000300009&script=sci_abstract&tlng=pt>. Accessed on: 12 Apr. 2016.

BEGHETTO, M.G.; *et al.* Nutritional assessment: description of the agreement between evaluators. *Rev Bras Epidemiol.* v.10, n.4, p.506-16, 2007.

BERBIGIER, M. C. *et al.* Bioelectrical impedance phase angle in septic patients admitted to intensive care units. *Rev Bras Ter Intensiva*, v. 25, n.1, p.25-31, 2013. Available at: <http://www.ncbi.nlm.nih.gov/pubmed/23887756>. Accessed on 12 Apr. 2016.

BLACKBURN, G. L.; BRISTIAN, B. R. Nutritional and metabolic assessment of the hospitalised patient. *JPEN.* v.1, p.11-22,1977.

BLUM D, *et al.* Cancer cachexia: a systematic literature review of items and domains associated with involuntary weight loss in cancer. *Crit Rev Oncol Hematol.* v.80, n.1, p.114-144, 2011.

BLUM, D. *et al.* Validation of the Consensus-Definition for Cancer Cachexia and evaluation of a classification model--a study based on data from an international multicentre project (EPCRC-CSA). *Ann Oncol.* v.25, n.8, p.1635-1642, 2014.

BONAMICHI, B.D.S.F. *et al.* Clinical applicability of glycated haemoglobin in the evolution of patients with hospital hyperglycemia. *Integr Mol Med.* v.2, n.4, p.248- 250, 2015.

BOSY-WESTPHAL, A. *et al.* Phase angle from bioelectrical impedance analysis: population reference values by age, sex, and body mass index. *JPEN J Parenter Enteral Nutr.* v.30, n.4, p.309-316, 2006.

BOTTONI, A. Nutritional assessment: laboratory tests. In: WAITZBERG, D. L. (ed.). *Oral, enteral and parenteral nutrition in clinical practice.* São Paulo: Atheneu, 2001. p.279-294.

BOZZETTI, F. *et al.* The nutritional risk in oncology: a study of 1,453 cancer outpatients. *Support Care Cancer.* v.20, p.1919-1928, 2012.

BRAZIL. Ministry of Health. *Food and Nutrition Surveillance* - SISVAN: basic guidelines for collecting, processing and analysing data and information in health services. Brasília:

Ministério da Saúde; 2004. (Series A. Normas e Manuais Técnicos). Disponívelem :
<http://189.28.128.100/nutricao/docs/geral/orientacoes_basicas_sisvan.pdf>.
HYPERLINK
"http://bvsms.saude.gov.br/bvs/publicacoes/orientacoes_basicas_sisvan.pdf.Acesso"
Accessed on: 11 Mar. 2016.

BRAUNSCHWEIG ,C.; GOMEZ, S.; SHEEAN, P.M. Impact of declines in nutritional status on outcomes in adult patients hospitalised for more than 7 days. *J Am Diet Assoc.* v. 100, n.11, p.1316-1322, 2000.

BROWNER, W. S.; CUMMINGS, S. R.; HULLEY, S. B. Estimating sample size and statistical power: basic points. In: HULLEY, S.B.; CUMMINGS, S.R. *Designing clinical research:* an epidemiological approach. Porto Alegre: Artmed, 2001. p.83-110.

BRUUN, L. I. *et al.* Prevalence of malnutrition in surgical patients: evaluation of nutritional support and documentation. *Clin Nutr.,* v. 18, n. 3, p.141-147, 1999.

BUDZIARECK, M. B.; DUARTE, R. R. P.; BARBOSA-SILVA, M. C. G Reference values and determinants for handgrip strength in healthy subjects. *Clinical Nutrition.* v.27, p.357-362, 2008.

CACCIALANZA, R. *et al.* Phase angle and handgrip strength are sensitive early markers of energy intake in hypophagic, non-surgical patients at nutritional risk, with contraindications to enteral nutrition. *Nutrients.* v.7, n.3, p.1828-1840, 2015.

CALAZANS, F. C. F. *et al.* Nutritional Screening in Surgical Patients in a University Hospital of Vitoria, ES, Brazil. *Nutr. clín. diet. hosp.* v. 35, n.3, p.34-41,2015.

CALIXTO-LIMA, L.; GONZALEZ, M. C. *Nutrição Clínica no dia a dia.* Rio de Janeiro: Rubio, 2013.

CARDINAL, T. R. *et al.* Standardised phase angle indicates nutritional status in hospitalized preoperative patients. *Nutr Res.* v.30, n.9, p.594-600, 2010.

CASTANHO, I. A. *et al.* Relationship between the phase angle and volume of tumours in patients with lung cancer. *Ann Nutr Metab.* v.62, n.1, p.68-74, 2013.

CATALANO, G. *et al.* The role of "bioelectrical impedance analysis" in the evaluation of the nutritional status of cancer patients. *Adv Exp Med Biol.* v.348, p.145-158,1993.

CERNE, D. *et al.* Lipoprotein lipase activity and gene expression in lung cancer and in adjacent non cancer lung tissue. *Exp Lung Res.* v.33, n.5, p. 217-225, 2007.

CHEN, C. H. *et al.* Hand-grip strength is a simple and effective outcome predictor in oesophageal cancer following oesophagectomy with reconstruction: a prospective study. *J Cardiothorac Surg.* v.6, n.98, p.1-5, 2011.

CHUMLEA, W. C. *et al.* Prediction of body weight for the nonambulatory elderly from anthropometry. *J Am Diet Assoc.* v.88, n.5, p.564-568, 1988.

CHUMLEA, W. C.; ROCHE, A. F.; STEINBAUGH, M. L. Estimating stature from knee height for persons 60 to 90 years of age. *J Am Geriatr Soc.* v.33, n.2, p. 116-120, 1985.

COLASANTO J. M. *et al.* Nutritional support of patients undergoing radiation therapy for head and neck cancer. *Oncology (Williston Park).* v.19, n.3, p.371-379, mar. 2005.

COOPER, R.; KUH, D.; HARDY, R. Objectively measured physical capability levels and mortality: systematic review and meta-analysis. *BMJ.* v.341, p.c4467, 2010.

COPPINI, L. Z.; WAITZBERG, D. L.; CAMPOS, A. C. Limitations and validation of bioelectrical impedance analysis in morbidly obese patients. *Curr Opin Clin Nutr Metab Care.* v.8, n.3, p.329-332, 2005.

CORREIA, M. I. T. D. Nutritional Assessment of Surgical Patients. In: CAMPOS, A. C. L. *Nutrição em Cirurgia.* São Paulo: Atheneu, 2001. p. 1-13.

CORREIA, M. I. T D. Subjective nutritional assessment. *Rev Bras Clin.* v. 13, p. 68-73, 1998.

CORREIA, M. I. T. Subjective global assessment: a reliable nutritional assessment tool to predict outcomes in critically ill patients. *Clinical nutrition* (Edinburgh, Scotland). v.33, n.2, p.291-295, 2014.

CORREIA, M. I. T.; CAMPOS, A. C. Prevalence of hospital malnutrition in Latin America: the multicentre ELAN study. *Nutrition.* v.19, n.10, p.823-825, 2003.

CORREIA, M.I.; WAITZBERG, D.L. The impact of malnutrition on morbidity, mortality, length of hospital stay and costs evaluated through a multivariate model analysis. *Clinical nutrition* (Edinburgh, Scotland). v.22, n.3, p.235-239, 2003.

COSTA, G. L. O. B. *Phase angle as an indicator of nutritional status in digestive tract cancer.* 2012. 92 f. Dissertation (Master's in Food, Nutrition and Health) - School of Nutrition, Federal University of Bahia; Salvador, 2012.

CUNNINGHAM, C.; LINDSEY, I. Colorectal cancer: management. *Colorectal Cancer,* v. 35, p.306-310, 2007.

CUSTEM, E.V.; ARENDS, J. The causes and consequences of cancer - associated malnutrition. *European Journal of Oncology Nursing,* v. 9, p. 51-63, 2005.

DAVIES, M. Nutritional screening and assessment in cancer-associated malnutrition. *Eur J Oncol Nurs.* v.9, Suppl 2, p.S64-73, 2005.

DELGADO-RODRÍGUEZ, M. *et al.* Cholesterol and serum albumin levels as predictors of cross infection, death, and length of hospital stay. *Arch Surg.* v. 137, n.7, p.805-812, 2002.

DETSKY, A. S. Nutritional status assessment: does it improve diagnostic or prognostic information. *Nutrition.* v. 7, n. 1, p.37-38, 1991.

DETSKY, A. S. *et al.* What is subjective global assessment of nutritional status? *JPEN J Parenter Enteral Nutr.* v. 11, n.1, p.8-13, 1987.

DETSKY, A.S.; *et al.* What is subjective global assessment of nutritional status? 1987. Classical article. *Nutr Hosp.* v. 23, n.4, p.400-407, 2008.

DEURENBERG, P. Invited commentary: Validation of body composition methods and assumptions. *Br J Nutr.* v. 90, p.485-486, 2003.

DEWYS, W. D. *et al.* Prognostic eff ect of weight loss prior to chemotherapy in cancer patients. Eastern Cooperative Oncology Group. *Am. J. Med.,* v. 69, n.4, p.491-497, 1980.

DUCHINI, L. *et al.* Assessment and monitoring of the nutritional status of hospitalised patients: a proposal based on the opinion of the scientific community. *Rev. Nutr.,* Campinas, v.23, n.4, p.513-522, Aug. 2010. Available at: <http://www.scielo.br/scielo.php?script=sci_arttext&pid=S1415- 52732010000400002>. Accessed on: 30 Apr. 2016.

DUERKSEN, D. R. *et al.* The validity and reproducibility of clinical assessment of nutritional status in the elderly. *Nutrition.* v.16, n.9, p.740-744, 2000.

DUVAL, P. A. *et al.* Cachexia in cancer patients admitted to an interdisciplinary home care programme. *Rev Bras Cancerologia..* v. 56, n.2, p.207- 212, 2010.

EHRMANN-JÓSKO, A. *et al.* Impaired glucose metabolism in colorectal cancer. *J. Scand J Gastroenterol.* v. 41, n. 9, p.1079-1086, Sep. 2006.

EICKEMBERG, M. *et al.* Electrical bioimpedance and its application in nutritional assessment. *Rev Nutr.,*Campinas. v.24, n.6, p.883-893, 2011. Available at: <http://www.scielo.br/scielo.php?script=sci_arttext&pid=S1415- 52732011000600009>. Accessed on: 02 Apr. 2016.

FEARON, K. *etal.* Definition_and_classification_of_cancer_cachexia: an_international_consensus. *Lancet Oncol.* v.12, n.5, p.489-495, 2011.

FEARON, K.C.; VOSS, A.C.; HUSTEAD, D.S. Definition of cancer cachexia: effect of weight loss, reduced food intake, and systemic inflammation on functional status and prognosis. *Am J Clin Nutr.* v.83, n.6, p.1345-1350, 2006.

FERNÁNDEZ, A. *et al.* Malnutrition in hospitalised patients receiving nutritionally complete menus: prevalence and outcomes. *Nutr Hosp.* v.30, n.6, p. 1344-1349, 2014.

FERREIRA, N. M. L.; SCARPA, A.; SILVA, D. A. Antineoplastic chemotherapy and nutrition: a complex relationship. *Revista Eletrónica de Enfermagem,* v.10, p.1026- 1034, 2008.

FLOOD, A. *et al.* The use of hand grip strength as a predictor of nutrition status in hospital patients. *Clin Nutr.* v.33, n.1, p.106-114, 2014.

FONTES, D. *Assessment of the nutritional status of critically ill patients.* 2011. 148f. Dissertation (Master's in Applied Sciences in Surgery and Ophthalmology) - School of Medicine, Federal University of Minas Gerais, Belo Horizonte, 2011.

FORCINA, D. V; ALMEIDA, B. O.; RIBEIRO JR, M. A F. Role of bariatric surgery in the control of type II diabetes mellitus. ***ABCD, arq. bras. cir. dig.*** v.21, n.3, p.130-132, 2008.

FRISANCHO, A. R. *Anthropometric Standards for the Assessment of Growth and Nutritional Status.* Ann Arbor, MI: The University of Michigan Press, 1990.

FRISANCHO, A. R.; FLEGEL, P. N. Relative merits of old and news indices of body mass with reference to skinfold thickness. *Am J Clin Nutr.,* v. 36, n.4, p.697-699, 1982.

FRISANCHO, A. R.Triceps skin fold and upper arm muscle size norms for assessment of nutrition status. *Am J Clin Nutr.* v.27, n.10, p.1052-1058, 1974.

GANEP Human Nutrition. *Physical Principles of Bioelectrical Impedance.* Course. Unravelling Bioelectrical Impedance in Clinical Practice Version 1.0.Lilian Mika Horie. GANEP: São Paulo, 2015. (Teaching material). Available at:

<http://www.ganepeducacao.com.br/>. Accessed on: 04 July 2015.

GOMES, P.M.; *et al.* Control of Intra-Hospital Hyperglycaemia in Critical and Non-Critical Patients. *Medicina.* Ribeirão Preto. v.47, n.2, p. 194-200, 2014. Available at: <http//:revista.fmrp.usp.br/>. Accessed on: 01 July 2015.

GONZALEZ, M.C. Subjective global assessment. In: WAITZBERG DL, editor. *Oral, enteral and parenteral nutrition in clinical practice.* 4.ed. São Paulo: Editora Atheneu, 2009. p. 341-371.

GRASSANI, S. G. *Diabetes x ICU.* Dissertation (Master's in Intensive Care Medicine) - Brazilian Intensive Care Medicine Association, Cuiabá, 2011.

GUERRA, M. R.; GALLO, C. V. M.; MENDONÇA, G A. S. Cancer risk in Brazil: trends and most recent epidemiological studies. *Rev Bras Cancerologia.* v. 51,

n. 3, p.227-234, 2005.

GUPTA, D. *et al.* Bioelectrical impedance phase angle in clinical practice: implications for prognosis in advanced colorectal cancer. *Am J Clin Nutr,* v. 80, n.6, p. 1634-1638, 2004a.

GUPTA, D.; *et al.* Bioelectrical impedance phase angle as a prognostic indicator in advanced pancreatic cancer. *Br J Nutr,* v. 92, n. 6, p. 957-962, 2004b.

GUPTA, D. *et al.* Bioelectrical impedance phase angle as a prognostic indicator in breast cancer. *BMC Cancer.* v. 8, n. 249, p.1-7, 2008.

GUPTA, D. *et al.* The relationship between bioelectrical impedance phase angle and subjective global assessment in advanced colorectal cancer. *Nutr J.,* v.7, n.19, p.1-6, 2009.

GUYTON, A. C.; HALL, J. E. *Treatise on medical physiology.* 10.ed. Rio de Janeiro: Guanabara Koogan, 2002.

HANLEY, J. A.; MC NEIL, B. J. A method of comparing the areas under receiver operating characteristic curves derived from the same cases. *Radiology.* v.148, n.3, p.839-843, sep.1983.

HEYMSFIELD, S. B. *et al.* Anthropometric measurements of muscle mass; revisited equation for calculating bone-free muscle area. *Am J Clin Nutr.* v. 36, n.4, p. 680-690, 1982.

HORIE, L. M. *et al.* New body fat prediction equations for severely obese patients. *Clin Nutr.* v. 27, n.3, p.350-356, 2008.

HORNBY, S. T. *et al.* Relationships between structural and functional measures of nutritional status in a normally nourished population. *Clin Nutr.* v.24, n.3, p.421-426, 2005.

HUI, D. *et al.* Phase angle for prognostication of survival in patients with advanced cancer: preliminary findings. *Cancer.* v.120, n.14, p.2207-2214, 2014.

HULLEY, S. B. *et al. Designing clinical research:* an epidemiologic approach. 2nded. Philadelphia: Lippincott Williams & Wilkins, 2001.

HUMPHREYS, J. *et al.* Muscle strength as a predictor of loss of functional status in hospitalised patients. *Nutrition*. v.18, n.8, p.616-620, 2002.

INCA. National Cancer Institute. *Brazilian Oncological Nutrition Survey.* Organised by Cristiane Aline D'Almeida, Nivaldo Barroso de Pinho. Rio de Janeiro: INCA, 2013.

INCA. National Cancer Institute. General Coordination of Strategic Actions. Prevention and Surveillance Coordination. *2014 estimate*: cancer incidence in Brazil. Rio de Janeiro: INCA, 2014.   124 p. Available at: <http://www1.inca.gov.br/vigilancia/>. Accessed on: 01 April 2014.

INCA. National Cancer Institute. General Coordination of Strategic Actions. Prevention and Surveillance Coordination. *2016/2017 estimate.* Rio de Janeiro: INCA, 2015b. Available at: <http://www.inca.gov.br/estimativa/2016/>. Accessed on: 01 April 2014.

INCA. National Cancer Institute. *Cancer treatment.* 2016. Available at: <http://www2.inca.gov.br/wps/wcm/connect/cancer/site/tratamento. Accessed on: 03 June 2016.

INCA. National Cancer Institute. *National Consensus on Oncological Nutrition.* Rio de Janeiro: INCA, 2009, 117p.

INCA. National Cancer Institute. General Coordination of Strategic Actions. Prevention and Surveillance Coordination. *National Cancer Institute* [homepage on the internet]. 2015a. Available at: <http://www.inca.gov.br>. Accessed on: 01 Dec. 2015.

INCA. National Cancer Institute. General Coordination of Strategic Actions. Prevention and Surveillance Coordination. *The cancer situation in Brazil.* Rio de Janeiro: INCA, 2008.   Available at   : <http://www.inca.gov.br/enfermagem/docs/cap1.pdf>. Accessed on: 10 October 2012.

IZAWA, K.P. *et al.* Handgrip strength as a predictor of prognosis in Japanese patients with congestive heart failure. *Eur J Cardiovasc Prev Rehabil.* v.16, n.1, p.21- 27, 2009.

JAMAR. *Hydraulic hand dynamometer owners manual.* Canada: Sammons Preston, 2000.   Available at   : <https://content.pattersonmedical.com/PDF/spr/Product/288115.pdf>. Accessed on: 10 Apr. 2016.

JANKOWSKA, R.; KOSACKA, M. Cancer cachexia syndrome in patients with lung cancer. *Wiad Lek,* v. 56, n.7-8, p.308-312, 2003.

JEEJEEBHOY, K. N. Nutritional assessment. *Gastroenterol Clin North Am.* v.27, n. 2, p. 347-369, 1998.

JEEJEEBHOY, K. N. Nutritional assessment. *Nutrition.* v.16, n.2, p.585, 2000.

JENSEN, G. L. *et al.* Recognising Malnutrition in Adults: definitions and Characteristics, Screening, Assessment, and Team Approach. *JPEN J Parenter Enteral Nutr.* v.37, p.802-807, 2013.

JENSEN, G.L.; *et al.* Adult starvation and disease-related malnutrition: a proposal for etiology-based diagnosis in the clinical practice setting from the International Consensus Guideline Committee .*JPEN J Parenter Enteral Nutr.* v.34, n.2, p.156-9. 2010.

JENSEN, G. L. *et al.* Malnutrition syndromes: a conundrum vs continuum. *JPEN J Parenter Enteral Nutr.* v.33, n.6, p.710-716, 2009.

JOSEP-ARGILÉS, M. J.; *et al.* Cancer cachexia: understanding the molecular basis. *Nat Rev Cancer*, v. 14, n. 11, p. 754-762, 2014.

KAISER, M. J. *et al.* Frequency of malnutrition in older adults: a multinational perspective using the mini nutritional assessment. *J Am Geriatr Soc.* v.58, n.9, p.1734-1738, 2010.

KAMIMURA, M. A. *et al.* Nutritional Assessment. In: CUPPARI, L. *Nutrição clínica no adulto.* Barueri, SP: Manole, 2005. p. 89-127.

KAVANAGH, B. P.; MCCOWEN, K. C. Clinical practice. Glycaemic control in the ICU. *N Engl J Med*, v. 363, n.26, p.2540-2546, 2010.

KLEE OEHLSCHLAEGER, M. H. *et al.* Nutritional status, muscle mass and strength of elderly in southern Brazil. *Nutr Hosp.* v.31, n.1, p.363-370, 2014.

KRAWCZYK, J. *et al.* Metabolic and nutritional aspects of cancer.*Postepy Hig Med Dosw.* v.68, n.2, p.1008-1014, 2014.

KVAMME, J.M. *et al.* Risk of malnutrition and zinc deficiency in community-living elderly men and women: the Troms0 Study. *Public Health Nutr.* v.18, n.11, p.1907- 1913, 2015.

KYLE, U. G. *et al.* Bioelectrical impedance analysis-part I: review of principles and methods. *Clin Nutr.* v.23, n.5, p.1226-1243, 2004a.

KYLE, U. G. *et al.* Can phase angle determined by bioelectrical impedance analysis assess nutritional risk? A comparison between healthy and hospitalised subjects. *Clin Nutr.,* v.31, n.6, p.875-881, 2012.

KYLE, U. G. *et al.* Body composition interpretation: contributions of the fat-free mass index and the body fat mass index. *Nutrition.* v.19, p.597-604, 2002.

KYLE, U. G. *et al.* Is nutritional depletion by nutritional risk index associated with increased length of hospital stay? A population based study. *JPEN.* v.28, n.2, p.99- 104, 2004b.

KYLE, U. G.; GENTON, L.; PICHARD, C. Hospital length of stay and nutritional status. *Curr Opin Clin Nutr Metab Care.* v.8, n.4, p.397-402. 2005.

KYLE, U. G.; GENTON, L.; PICHARD, C. Low phase angle determined by bioelectrical impedance analysis is associated with malnutrition and nutritional risk at hospital admission. *Clin Nutr.* v.32, n.2, p.294-299, 2013.

LANDIS, J. R.; KOCH, G. G. The measurement of observer agreement for categorical data. *Biometrics.* v.33, n.1, p.159-174, Mar.1977.

LEANDRO-MERHI, A. *et al.* Comparative study of nutritional indicators in patients with neoplasms of the digestive tract. *Brazilian Archives of Digestive Surgery.* v. 21, n.3, p.114-119, 2008.

LEITE, S. A. *et al.* Impact of hyperglycemia on morbidity and mortality, length of hospitalisation and rates of re-hospitalization in a general hospital setting in Brazil. *Diabetol Metab Syndr.* v.2, n.1, p.49, 2010.

LIMA, K. V. G.; MAIO R. Nutritional status, systemic inflammation and prognosis of patients with gastrointestinal cancer. *Nutr Hosp.* v.27, n.3, p.707-714, 2012.

LIMBERGER, V. R.; PASTORE, C. A.; ABIB, R. T. Association between hand dynamometry, nutritional status and postoperative complications in oncological patients. *Revista Brasileira de Cancerologia.* v.60, n.2, p. 135-141, 2014. Available at: <http://www.inca.gov.br/rbc/n_60/v02/pdf/07-artigo-associacao-entre- dynamometria-manual-estado-nutricional-and-complicacoes-pos-operatorias-em- pacientes-oncologicos.pdf.> Accessed on: 24 July 2016.

LLAMES, L. *et al.* Phase angle values by electrical bioimpedance: nutritional status and prognostic value. *Nutr Hosp.,* Madrid. v.28, n.2, p.286-295, 2013. Available at: <http://scielo.isciii.es/scielo.php?script=sci_arttext&pid=S0212-16112013000200004&lng=es&nrm=iso>. Accessed on: 12 Apr. 2016.

LLOVET, J. M. Hepatocellular carcinoma .*Lancet.* v.362, n.9399, p.1907-1917, 2003.

LOHMAN, T G. *Advances in body composition assessment* - current issues in exercise science series. Champaing: Human Kinetics, 1992.

LOHMAN, T G.; ROCHE, A. F.; MARTORELL, R. *Anthropometrics Standardisation Reference Manual.* Illinois: Human Kinetics Book, 1988.

LUCAS, M. C. S.; FAYH, A. P. T Nutritional status, hyperglycaemia, early nutrition and mortality of patients admitted to an intensive care unit. *Rev. bras. ter. intensiva,* São Paulo, v.24, n.2, p.157-161, jun. 2012. Available at: <http://www.scielo.br/scielo.php?script=sci_arttext&pid=S0103-507X2012000200010&lng=en&nrm=iso>. Accessed on: 01 April 2016.

MAGGIORE, Q. *et al.* Nutritional and prognostic correlates of bioimpedance indexes in haemodialysis patients. *Kidney Int.* v.50, n.6, p.2103-2108, 1996.

MALECKA-MASSALSKA, T *et al.* Bioelectrical impedance phase angle and subjective global assessment in detecting malnutrition among newly diagnosed head and neck cancer patients. *Eur Arch Otorhinolaryngol.* v.273, n.5, p.1299-1305, 2015.

MARIN CARO, M. M. *et al* . Evaluation of nutritional risk and establishment of nutritional support in oncological patients, according to the protocol of the Spanish Nutrition and Cancer Group. *Nutr. Hosp.* Madrid. v.23, n.5, p.458-468, oct., 2008.
Available at: <http://scielo.isciii.es/scielo.php?script=sci_arttext&pid=S0212-16112008000700008&lng=es&nrm=iso>. Accessed on: 22 May 2016.

MARTÍNEZ OLMOS, M. A. *et al.* Nutritional status study of inpatients in hospitals of Galicia. *Eur J Clin Nutr.* v.59, n.8, p.938-946, 2005.

MARTINS, C. Body composition and muscle function. In: MARTINS, C. *Avaliação do Estado Nutricional e Diagnóstico.* São Paulo: Nutroclinica, 2008. p. 245-286.

MAULDIN, K.; O'LEARY-KELLEY, C. New Guidelines for Assessment of Malnutrition in Adults: Obese Critically Ill Patients. *Crit Care Nurse.* v.35, n.4, p.24-30, 2015.

MELSTROM, L. G. *et al.* Mechanisms of skeletal muscle degradation and its therapy in cancer cachexia. Histol *Histopathol.* v.22, n.7, p.805-814, 2007.

MEYER, F. J. *et al.* Respiratory muscle dysfunction in congestive heart failure: clinical correlation and prognostic significance. *Circulation.* v.103, n.17, p.2153-2158, 2001.

MONTANO-LOZA, A. J. *et al.* Inclusion of Sarcopenia within MELD (MELD- sarcopenia) and the prediction of mortality in patients with cirrhosis. *Clin Transl Gastroenterol.* v.6, S n , p e102, 2015.

MONTEIRO, C. A. *et al.* Causes of the decline in child malnutrition in Brazil, 19962007. *Rev. Saúde Pública*, São Paulo , v. 43, n. 1, p.35-43, feb. 2009. Available at: <http://www.scielo.br/pdf/rsp/v43n1/498.pdf>. Accessed on: 12 Apr. 2016.

MOREIRA, D. *et al.* Approach to palmar grip using the Jamar dynamometer: a literature review. *R.   Bras.   Ci.   e   Mov.*   Brasília,   v.11,   n.2,   p.95-99,   2003. Available at   : <http://portalrevistas.ucb.br/index.php/RBCM/article/viewFile/502/527>. Accessed on: 09 October 2015.

MORIN, P. J. *et al.* Cancer Genetics. In: KASPER, D.L. *et al. Harrison Internal Medicine.* 17.ed. Rio de Janeiro: McGraw-Hill interamericana do Brasil, 2008. p.468- 474.

MOTTA, R. S. T.; CASTANHO, I. A.; VELARDE, L. G. C. Valoración nutricional Cutoff point of the phase angle in pre-radiotherapy cancer patients. *Nutr Hosp.* v.32, n.5, p.2253-2260, 2015.

MUSSOI, T D. *Assessment of nutritional status in clinical practice*: from pregnancy to ageing. Rio de Janeiro: Guanabara Koogan, 2014.

NAGANO, M.; SUITA, S.; YAMANOUCHI, T. The validity of bioelectrical impedance phase angle for nutritional assessment in children. *J Pediatr Surg.* v.35, n.7, p.1035-1039, 2000.

NICE-SUGAR STUDY INVESTIGATORS *et al.* Intensive versus conventional glucose control in critically ill patients. *N Engl J Med.* v.360, n.13, p.1283-1297, 2009.

NORMAN, K. *et al.* Bioimpedance vector analysis as a measure of muscle function. *Clin. Nutr.* v.28, n., p.78-82, 2009.

NORMAN, K. *et al.* Cutoff percentiles of bioelectrical phase angle predict functionality, quality of life, and mortality in patients with cancer. *Am J Clin Nutr.* v.92, n.3, p.612-619, 2010.

NORMAN, K. *et al.* Effects of creatine supplementation on nutritional status, muscle function and quality of life in patients with colorectal cancer - a double blind randomised controlled trial. *Clin Nutr.* v. 25, n.4, p.596-605, 2006.

NORMAN, K. *et al.* Hand grip strength: outcome predictor and marker of nutritional status. *Clin Nutr.* v.30, n.2, p.135-142, 2011.

NURSAL, T. Z. *et al.* Simple two-part tool for screening of malnutrition. *Nutrition.* v.21, p.659-665, 2005.

OLIVEIRA, P. G. *Phase Angle as an Indicator of Negative Outcomes in Surgical Patients.* 2012. 81 f. Dissertation (Master's in Medicine) - School of Medicine, Universidade Federal do Rio Grande do Sul; Porto Alegre, 2012.

OTTERY, F. D. Definition of standardised nutritional assessment and interventional pathways in oncology. *Nutrition.* v.12, n.1, Suppl.1, p.S15-S19, jan. 1996.

PABLO, A. M.; IZAGA, M. A.; ALDAY, L. A. Assessment of nutritional status on hospital admission: nutritional scores. *Eur J Clin Nutr.,* v. 57, n.7, p.824-831,2003.

PAIVA, S. I. *Use of bioimpedance to monitor chemotherapy patients:* changes in phase angle. 2007. 50f. Dissertation (Master's in Health and Behaviour) - School of Psychology and School of Health, Catholic University of Pelotas, Pelotas, 2007.

PAIVA, S. I. *et al.* Standardised phase angle from bioelectrical impedance analysis as prognostic factor for survival in patients with cancer. *Support Care Cancer.* v.19, n.2, p.187-192, 2010.

PAIXÃO, E. M.; GONZALEZ, M. C.; ITO, M. K. A prospective study on the radiation therapy associated changes in body weight and bioelectrical standardised phase angle. *Clin Nutr.* v.34, n.3, p.496-500, 2015.

PAN, H. *et al.* The impact of nutritional status, nutritional risk, and nutritional treatment on clinical outcome of 2248 hospitalised cancer patients: a multi-center, prospective cohort study in Chinese teaching hospitals. *Nutr Cancer.* v.65, n.1, p.62- 70, 2013.

PASTORES, C. A.; OEHLSCHALAEGER, M. H. K.; GONZALEZ, M. C. Impact of Nutritional Status and Muscle Strength on Global Health and Quality of Life Status in Gastrointestinal and Lung Cancer Patients. *Rev. bras. Cancerol.* v.59, n.1, p.43-49, 2013. Available at: <http://www.inca.gov.br/rbc/n_59/v01/pdf/07-impacto-do- estado-nutricional-e-da-for%C3%A7a-muscular.pdf>. Accessed on: 12 Apr. 2016.

PENNIÉ, J. B. State of malnutrition in Cuban hospitals. *Nutrition.* v.21, p.487-497, 2005.

PERES, W. A. *et al.* Phase angle as a nutritional evaluation tool in all stages of chronic liver disease. *Nutr Hosp.* v.27, n.6, p.2072-2078, 2012.

PIRLICH, M. *et al.* Social risk factors for hospital malnutrition. *Nutrition.* v.21, p.295- 300, 2005.

PUPIM, L. B. *et al.* Uremic malnutrition is a predictor of death independent of inflammatory status. *Kidney Int.* v.66, n.5, p.2054-2060, 2004.

RANTANEN, T. *et al.* Handgrip strength and cause-specific and total mortality in older disabled women: exploring the mechanism. *J Am Geriatr Soc.* v.51, n.5, p.636- 641,2003.

RAVASCO, P. *et al.* Impact of nutrition on outcome: a prospective randomised controlled trial in patients with head and neck cancer undergoing radiotherapy. *Head Neck.* v.27, n.8, p.659-668, 2005.

RECH, C. R. *et al.* Validity of anthropometric equations for estimating body fat in elderly people in southern Brazil. *Rev. bras. cineanthropom. desempenho hum.* Florianópolis, v.12, n.1, p.01-07, feb. 2010.

RJL SYSTEM. *Quantum II & Quantum X Bioelectrical Impedance Analysers.* Available at: <http://www.rjlsystems.com/support/docs/analyzers/quantum iix/Quantum_IIX_Manual.pdf. Accessed on: 08 October 2015.

RODRIGUES, R. C. Quality Control Committee. Intensive Care Sector - UNIFESP. *Glycaemic Control Protocol.* São Paulo: UNIFESP, 2008. Available at: <http://www.saudedireta.com.br/docsupload/1339871979controle_glicemico.pdf>. Accessed on: 01 July 2015.

RUBINO F. *et al.* The Early Effect of the Roux-en-Y Gastric Bypass on Hormones Involved in Body Weight Regulation and Glucose Metabolism. *Ann Surg.* v.1, n.240, p.236-242, 2004.

RUIZ-MARGÁIN, A. *et al.* Malnutrition assessed through phase angle and its relation to prognosis in patients with compensated liver cirrhosis: a prospective cohort study. *Dig Liver Dis.* v.47, n.4, p.309-314, 2015.

RYU, T Y.; PARK, J.; SCHERER, P. E. Hyperglycaemia as a Risk Factor for Cancer Progression. *Diabetes Metab J.* v.38, n.5, p.330-336, 2014.

SACKS, D. B. *et al.* Guidelines and recommendations for laboratory analysis in the diagnosis and management of diabetes mellitus. *Diabetes Care.* v.25, p.750-786, 2003.

SALLINEN J. *et al.* Hand-grip strength cut-points to screen older persons at risk for mobility limitation. *J Am Geriatr Soc.* v.58, n.9, p.1721-1726, 2010.

SAMPAIO, M. R. M.; PINTO, F. J. M.; VASCONCELOS, C. M. C. S. Nutritional assessment of hospitalised patients: agreement between different methods. *Rev Bras Promoç Saúde.* v.25, n.1, p. 110-115, 2012. Available at: <http://www.redalyc.org/pdf/408/40823228016.pdf>. Accessed on: 15 Apr. 2016.

SCHEUNEMANN, L. *et al.* Agreement and association between the phase angle and parameters of nutritional status assessment in surgical patients. *Nutr Hosp.* v.26, n.3, p.480-487, 2011.

SCHLUSSEL, M. M.; ANJOS, L. A.; KAC, G Hand grip strength test and its use in nutritional assessment. *Rev. Nutr.,* Campinas, v.21, n.2, p. 223-235, 2008.
Available from:<http://www.scielo.br/scielo.php?pid=S1415-
52732008000200009&script=sci_abstract>. Accessed on: 12 Apr. 2016.

SCHLUSSEL, M. M. *et al.* Referente values of handgrip dynamometry of health adults: A populatin-based study. *Clin Nutr.* v. 27, n.4, p.601-607, 2008.

SCHRAIBER, L.B. *et al.* Health needs and masculinities: primary care for men. *Cad. Saúde Pública.* v.26, n.5, p.961-970, 2010.

SCHUTTE, K.; SCHULZ, C.; MALFERTHEINER, P. Nutrition and Hepatocellular Cancer. *Gastrointest Tumours.* v.2, p. 188-194, 2015. Available at: <http://www.karger.com/Article/PDF/441822>. Accessed on: 04 May 2016.

SELBERG ,O.; SELBERG, D. Norms and correlates of bioimpedance phase angle in healthy human subjects, hospitalised patients, and patients with liver cirrhosis. *Eur J Appl Physiol.* v.86, n.6, p.509-516, 2002.

SILVA ,T K. *et al.* Phase angle as a prognostic marker in patients with critical illness. *Nutr Clin Pract.* v.30, n.2, p.:261-265, 2015.

SILVA, L. M. D. L.; CARUSO, L.; MARTINI, L. A. Application of the phase angle in clinical situations. *Revista Brasileira de Nutrição Clinica.* v.22, n.4, p.317-321,2007.

SILVA, M. C. G. B. *Use of subjective nutritional assessment and bioimpedance as prognostic factors for post-operative complications in digestive tract surgeries.* 2002. 222f. Thesis (Doctorate in Epidemiology) - Federal University of Pelotas, Pelotas, 2002.

SLEE, A.; BIRCH, D; STOKOE, D. Bioelectrical impedance vector analysis, phase- angle assessment and relationship with malnutrition risk in a cohort of frail older hospital patients in the United Kingdom. *Nutrition,* v. 31, n.1, p.132-137, 2015.

SMITH, L. C.; MULLEN, J. L. Nutritional assessment and indications for nutritional support.*Surg Clin North Am.* v.71, n.3, p.449-457, 1991.

BRAZILIAN DIABETES SOCIETY (SBD). *D635 Brazilian Diabetes Society Guidelines:* 2014-2015/Brazilian Diabetes Society. São Paulo: AC Farmacêutica, 2015b.

BRAZILIAN DIABETES SOCIETY (SBD). *Brazilian Diabetes Society Guidelines:* 2013-2014. São Paulo: AC Farmacêutica, 2014. Available at: <http://www.nutritotal.com.br/diretrizes/files/342--diretrizessbd.pdf>. Accessed on: 12 Apr. 2016.

BRAZILIAN DIABETES SOCIETY (SBD). *SBD Official Positioning n⁰ 03/2015*: glycaemic control in hospitalised patients. São Paulo: SBD, 2015a.

SOTELO GONZALEZ, S. *et al.* Anthropometric parameters in the evaluation of malnutrition in hospitalised cancer patients: use of body mass index and weight loss percentage. *Nutr. Hosp.* Madrid, v.28, n.3, p.965- 968, jun. 2013. Available at : <http://scielo.isciii.es/scielo.php?script=sci_arttext&pid=S0212-16112013000300057&lng=es&nrm=iso>. Accessed on: 22 May 2016.

STEENSON, J.; VIVANTI, A.; ISENRING, E. Inter-rater reliability of the Subjective Global Assessment: a systematic literature review. *Nutrition.* v.29, n.1, p.350-352, 2013.

STEGEL, P. *et al.* Bioelectrical impedance phase angle as an indicator and predictor of cachexia in head and neck cancer patients treated with (chemotherapy) radiotherapy. *Eur J Clin Nutr.* v.1, S.n, feb., 2016.

THOMAS, M. B. Liver tumours. In: HOFF, P. M. G. *et al.* (Ed.). *Treatise on oncology.* São Paulo: Atheneu, 2013. p.120.

TOSO, S. *et al.* Altered tissue electrical properties in lung cancer patients as detected by bioelectric impedance vector analysis. *Nutrition.* v.16, n.2, p.120-124, 2000.

UMPIERREZ, G. E. *et al.* Hyperglycemia: an independent marker of in-hospital mortality in patients with undiagnosed diabetes. *J Clin Endocrinol Metab.* v.87, n.3, p.978-982, 2002.

VAN DEN BERGHE, G. *et al.* Intensive insulin therapy in critically ill patients. *N Engl J Med,* v.345, n.19, p.1359-1367, 2001.

VAN DEN BERGHE, G. *et al.* Intensive insulin therapy in the medical ICU. *N Engl J Med.* v.354, n.5, p.449-461,2006.

VANNUCHI, H.; UNAMUNO, M. R. D. L.; MARCHINI, J. S. Evaluation of nutritional status. *Medicina* (Ribeirão Preto). v.29, n.1, p.5-18, 1996. Available at: <http://www.revistas.usp.br/rmrp/article/view/707/719>. Accessed on: 12 Apr. 2012.

VICENTE, M. *et al.* What are the most effective methods for assessment of nutritional status in outpatients with gastric and colorectal cancer? *Nutr Hosp.* v.28, n.3, p.585-591,2013.

VIGANO, A. *et al.* Clinical survival predictors in patients with advanced cancer. *Arch. Intern. Med.,* v.160, n.6, p.861-868, 2000.

WAITZBERG, D. L.; CAIAFFA, W. T.; CORREIA, M. I. Hospital malnutrition: the brazilian national survey (IBRANUTRI): a study of 4000 patients. *Nutrition.* v.17, n.7-8, p.573-580, 2001.

WAITZBERG, D. L. *Oral, Enteral and Parenteral Nutrition in Clinical Practice*. 3.ed. São Paulo: Atheneu Publishing House, 2004.

WAITZBERG, D. L.; CORREIA, M. I. Nutritional assessment in the hospitalised patient. *Curr Opin Clin Nutr Metab Care*. v.6, n.5, p.531-538, 2003.

WESTPHAL, A. *et al*. Phase angle from bioelectrical impedance analysis: Population reference values by age, sex, and body mass index. *JPEN J Parenter Enteral Nutr* v.30, p.309-316, 2006.

WHITE, J. V. *et al*. Consensus statement of the Academy of Nutrition and Dietetics/American Society for Parenteral and Enteral Nutrition: characteristics recommended for the identification and documentation of adult malnutrition (undernutrition). *J Acad Nutr Diet*. v.112, n.5, p.730-738, 2012a.

WHITE, J. V. *et al*. Consensus statement: Academy of Nutrition and Dietetics and American Society for Parenteral and Enteral Nutrition: characteristics recommended

for the identification and documentation of adult malnutrition (undernutrition). *JPEN J Parenter Enteral Nutr*. v.36, n.3, p.275-283, 2012b.

WILHELM-LEEN, E. R. *et al*. Phase angle, frailty and mortality in older adults. *J Gen Intern Med*. v.29, n.1, p.147-154, 2014.

WORLD HEALTH ORGANISATION (WHO). *WHO Expert Committee on Physical Status: The use and Interpretation of Anthropometry*. Geneva: World Health Organisation, 1995 (WHO technical report series; 854). Available at: <http://apps.who.int/iris/bitstream/10665/37003/1/WHO_TRS_854.pdf>. Accessed on: 05 Apr. 2016.

YEON LEE, *et al*. Phase Angle and Survival Time in Terminal Cancer. *J Med*. v.35, n.05, Sep., 2014.

APPENDICES

APPENDIX A - INFORMED CONSENT FORM

Dear Sir or Madam,____

You are being invited to take part in the research project "Phase angle associated with the nutritional and hydration status of patients with malignant neoplasms undergoing surgical treatment". The aim of the study is to assess the relationship between the phase angle (which is a value given when assessing body composition using an electrical bioimpedance device, in which an electric current passes that cannot be felt and therefore does not hurt) and the health of patients with a lesion in any part of the head, neck or digestive tract who have been hospitalised for surgery. Your participation is voluntary and there are no risks or harm to your treatment. You will not suffer any discrimination or harm to your treatment if you do not wish to take part in the research or if you withdraw your consent at any time during the study. Your participation consists of allowing information from your medical records about your illness to be used in the research. In addition, a nutritional assessment will be carried out four times, consisting of body measurements (such as weight, height and circumferences), body composition (amount of fat and muscle in the body), muscle strength and capillary glycaemia using a device called a glucometer. The information in this survey is confidential and your identity will not be revealed. The information will only be used for the research. You have complete freedom to clarify any doubts that may arise before and during the course of the research.

I have read and understood the above information and agree to voluntarily participate in the project.

Belo Horizonte, 2015.

Name and registration number	Participant's signature
Name	Student's signature
Name	Researcher's signature

Natália Fenner (Master's student) - (31) 93187048/natalia.fenner@hotmail.com
Simone Generoso (Researcher) (31) 8812-8650/simonenutufmg@gmail.com
Research Ethics Committee, UFMG (31) 3409-4592Av. Antônio Carlos, 6627 - Unidade Administrative II - 2nd floor - Room 2005

APPENDIX B - DATA COLLECTION INSTRUMENT

PROJECT: AF - UFMG/HC - INSTITUTO ALFA . RESPONSIBLE FOR

COMPLETION: _______________________________

---

1)   Identification

Medical record number: No. ot bed ___________
Name: Contact: (____) -

Sex: (1   ) Female   (2   )   Male
Proceedings: _______________________________
Race: Age:

Marital **status**: (1) Single (2) Married / civil partnership (3) Widowed (4) Divorced
Date of birth   /___/Date of hospitalisation:_______//

---

2)   Health History

Local tumour: (1) EED (2) CCP (3) COLOP (4) FVB
Type of tumour: _______________________________
Time since diagnosis: years months.
Type of patient treatment: (1) Surgical
Previous history: (1) SAH (2) DM (3) CRF (4) Dyslipidaemia (5) AMI (6) CHF(7) Stroke
(8)   Other,   which one   (s)
                          ?

---

3)   Nutritional Assessment

A) Subjective Global Assessment (SGA)
History

Weight
Usual weight: Kg. % PP:
Have you lost weight in the last 6 months? (1) Yes (2) No (3) Unknown Amount lost: Kg.
In the last 2 weeks: (1) Still losing (2) Stable (3) Put on weight
Food intake compared to usual
(1) No changes (2) there were changes.
If so, how long ago: days.
If any, for diet: (1) Solid, smaller quantity (2) Complete liquid (3) Restricted liquid (4)
Fasting
Gastrointestinal symptoms present for more than 15 days
(1) Yes (2) No
Lack of appetite: (1) Yes (2) No Nausea: (1) Yes (2) No Vomiting: (1) Yes (2) No
Diarrhoea - More than 3 liquid bowel movements per day: (1) Yes (2) No
Functional capacity
(1) Without dysfunction (2) With dysfunction
If changed, how long ago: days.
Type of dysfunction: (1) Suboptimal work (2) Outpatient treatment (3) Bedridden Main
illness and its relationship to nutritional needs Main diagnosis(es): __________
Metabolic demand: (1) Low stress (2) Moderate stress (3) High stress

Physical examination
Give each item a value:

0 = Normal	____	Loss of subcutaneous fat (triceps and chest)
1 = Light	____	Muscle loss (quadriceps and deltoid)
2 = Moderate	____	Presence of malleolar oedema
3 = Important	____	Presence of presacral oedema

Subjective evaluation
Final results:
(1) Nourished (2) Suspected malnutrition or moderately malnourished (3) Severely
malnourished
2 Classifications
(1) Eutrophic (2) Malnourished Source: Detsky *et al.*,(1987).

Biochemical Test

Variable	PO/Inpatient OR 24h PO//	Between 3rd and 5th DPO//	Hospital Discharge //
Blood sugar 06h00min 18.00	-	-	-

Anthropometry   Estimated date of ________________ surgery
   / /

Variable	PO Hospitalisation //	24h PO //	Between 3rd and 5th DPO //	Hospital Discharge //
Current weight (kg)				
Height (m)				
Circumference Handle (cm)				
ComplexionSmallMediumLarge Bone				
CB (cm)				

Classification CB (1) with deficit (2) without deficit				
PCT (cm)				
PCT classification (1) with deficit (2) without deficit				
CMB				
AMB				
AMB classification (1) with deficit (2) without deficit				
BMI				
Classification BMI (1) Nourished (2) Malnourished				

RESPONSIBLE FOR FULFILMENT ____

Functional Assessment

Variable	PO Hospitalisation //	24h PO //	Between 3rd and 5th DPO //	Hospital Discharge //
Dynamometry (1) Right (2) Left	Average	Average	Average	Average ________

Ob: Position/arm > Angle = 90°; Check that the patient has access and mark "X" on the dominant arm

Electrical bioimpedance

Variable	PO Hospitalisation //	24h PO //	Between 3rd and 5th DPO //	Hospital Discharge //
Resistance				
Reactance				
Fat-free mass (kg)				
Body fat percentage				
Total body water				
Phase angle				

4) Clinical outcome

Postoperative infectious and non-infectious complications

Variable	Presence	Variable	Presence
Wound infection	(1) Yes (2) No	Surgical wound dehiscence	(1) Yes (2) No
Abdominal abscess	(1) Yes (2) No	Blood transfusion	(1) Yes (2) No
Pneumonia	(1) Yes (2) No	Acute respiratory failure	(1) Yes (2) No
Urinary tract infection	(1) Yes (2) No	Renal insufficiency	(1) Yes (2) No
Bacteraemia	(1) Yes (2) No	Cardiocirculatory insufficiency	(1) Yes (2) No
Venous catheter infection	(1) Yes (2) No	Liver dysfunction	(1) Yes (2) No
Sepsis	(1) Yes (2) No	Fistula	(1) Yes (2) No

Use of antibiotics during hospitalisation: (1) Yes (2) No

Length of stay: ICU _______________ Total post-operative: ___________

Date of hospital discharge: // ___ Death: (1) Yes (2) No

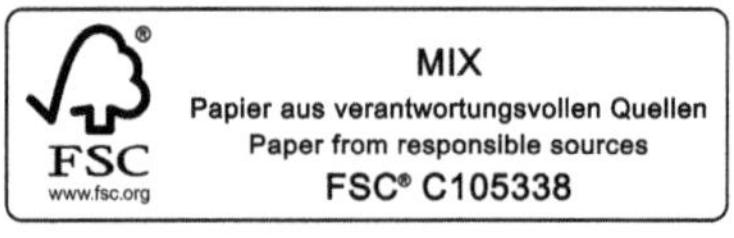

Printed by Books on Demand GmbH, Norderstedt / Germany